Bioemergency Planning

Angela Hewlett • A. Rekha K. Murthy
Editors

Bioemergency Planning

A Guide for Healthcare Facilities

Springer

Editors
Angela Hewlett
Division of Infectious Diseases
Nebraska Biocontainment Unit
University of Nebraska Medical Center
Omaha, NE, USA

A. Rekha K. Murthy
Division of Infectious Diseases
Department of Medical Affairs
Cedars-Sinai Medical Center
Los Angeles, CA, USA

ISBN 978-3-319-77031-4 ISBN 978-3-319-77032-1 (eBook)
https://doi.org/10.1007/978-3-319-77032-1

Library of Congress Control Number: 2018940499

Printed on acid-free paper

This Springer imprint is published by the registered company Springer International Publishing AG part of Springer Nature.
The registered company address is: Gewerbestrasse 11, 6330 Cham, Switzerland

Dedicated to all the heroes: Patients and families who have experienced the devastation of the Ebola epidemic and to the courage and dedication of all the healthcare professionals, first responders, researchers, and volunteers who risk their lives to protect their patients and the public.

"Courage is not the absence of fear, but rather the judgment that something else is more important than one's fear."

Ambrose Hollingworth Redmoon, *from No Peaceful Warriors*

Preface

Preparing a healthcare facility to care for patients with known or suspected highly hazardous communicable diseases requires significant effort and can be a daunting task. This was well illustrated in 2014, when healthcare facilities around the world rapidly developed and augmented preparedness plans in response to the outbreak of Ebola virus disease in West Africa. These efforts were accompanied by significant challenges, many of which were unanticipated, along with a paucity of clear guidance on issues encountered. This resulted in many lessons learned.

We chose to use our experience during and following the 2014–2016 Ebola outbreak to create *Bioemergency Planning: A Guide for Healthcare Facilities*. The intent of this book is to discuss the challenges we and countless others faced, as well as transparently share the lessons learned from healthcare facilities around the world. The authors of the chapters in this book were selected to share their expertise based on their real-world experience in hospital preparedness. Chapters include a wide variety of preparedness topics, from designing a biocontainment space to creating and maintaining a multidisciplinary patient care team. Many of the chapters address topics that presented major challenges in preparedness, including decontamination and waste management, safe and comprehensive laboratory analysis, patient transport, and the care of the deceased patient. Caring for special populations, including pregnant women and pediatric patients, deserves attention due to the unique issues involved, and these topics are addressed in dedicated chapters by experts in the field. Chapters on behavioral health, media and communications, regulatory issues, administrative support, and research were included since preplanning can mitigate some of the difficulties in navigating these often complex topics in preparedness.

All healthcare facilities, from the smallest critical access hospital to the largest tertiary care center, must be prepared to identify, isolate, and provide care for patients with suspected or confirmed highly hazardous communicable diseases. Although it is easy to become complacent once an outbreak subsides and is no longer in the headlines, we must remain vigilant in order to be prepared for the next outbreak, whether it is Ebola, influenza, or a novel pathogen not yet discovered. It is our hope that this book will serve as a practical guide for healthcare facilities to enhance preparedness efforts.

Omaha, NE, USA — Angela Hewlett, MD, MS
Los Angeles, CA, USA — A. Rekha K. Murthy, MD

Contents

Editors and Contributors

Editors

Angela Hewlett, MD, MS Associate Professor, Division of Infectious Diseases, Medical Director, Nebraska Biocontainment Unit, University of Nebraska Medical Center, Omaha, NE, USA

A. Rekha K. Murthy, MD Professor of Medicine, Division of Infectious Diseases, Vice President for Medical Affairs and Associate Chief Medical Officer, Cedars-Sinai Medical Center and Professor of Clinical Medicine, David Geffen School of Medicine at UCLA, Los Angeles, CA, USA

Contributors

Roxanne Alter, BSMT, MS Nebraska Public Health Laboratory, Department of Pathology and Microbiology, University of Nebraska Medical Center, Omaha, NE, USA

Amy S. Arrington, MD, PhD Medical Director, Pediatric Special Isolation Unit, Pediatric Critical Care Medicine, Texas Children's Hospital, Baylor College of Medicine, Houston, TX, USA

Paul D. Biddinger, MD Vice Chairman for Emergency Preparedness, Department of Emergency Medicine, Director, Center for Disaster Medicine, Director, Region 1 Ebola and Other Special Pathogens Treatment Center, Massachusetts General Hospital, Boston, MA, USA

Kate Boulter, RN, MPH The Nebraska Biocontainment Unit, Nebraska Medicine, Omaha, NE, USA

Nicholas V. Cagliuso Sr., PhD, MPH Senior Assistant, Vice President for Emergency Management, Office of the President & CEO, NYC Health + Hospitals, New York, NY, USA

David S. Cates, PhD Director of Behavioral Health, Nebraska Medicine/ University of Nebraska Medical Center, Omaha, NE, USA

Theodore J. Cieslak, MD The Nebraska Biocontainment Unit, Department of Epidemiology, College of Public Health, University of Nebraska Medical Center, Omaha, NE, USA

Jared D. Evans, PhD Department of Emergency Medicine, Johns Hopkins University, Baltimore, MD, USA

Research and Exploratory Development Department, Johns Hopkins University Applied Physics Laboratory, Laurel, MD, USA

Brian T. Garibaldi, MD Medical Director, Johns Hopkins Biocontainment Unit, Pulmonary and Critical Care, Johns Hopkins University School of Medicine, Baltimore, MD, USA

Paula G. Gomes, PsyD Faculty Staff Assistance Program, Emory University, Atlanta, GA, USA

Bruce Gordon, MD Executive Chair, Institutional Review Board, University of Nebraska Medical Center, Omaha, NE, USA

Vicki L. Herrera, MS Nebraska Public Health Laboratory, Department of Pathology and Microbiology, University of Nebraska Medical Center, Omaha, NE, USA

Jocelyn J. Herstein, MPH Department of Environmental, Agricultural & Occupational Health, College of Public Health, University of Nebraska Medical Center, Omaha, NE, USA

Steven H. Hinrichs, MD Medical Director, Nebraska Public Health Laboratory, Department of Pathology and Microbiology, University of Nebraska Medical Center, Omaha, NE, USA

John P. Horton, MD Department of Gynecology and Obstetrics, Division of General Obstetrics and Gynecology, Emory University Healthcare, Atlanta, GA, USA

Jordan A. Hughes, MHA Department of Medicine, Johns Hopkins Hospital, Baltimore, MD, USA

Alexander P. Isakov, MD, MPH Section of Prehospital and Disaster Medicine, Department of Emergency Medicine, Emory University School of Medicine, Atlanta, GA, USA

Peter C. Iwen, MS, PhD, D(ABMM) Laboratory Director, Nebraska Public Health Laboratory, Department of Pathology and Microbiology, University of Nebraska Medical Center, Omaha, NE, USA

Katelyn Jelden, MPH College of Medicine, University of Nebraska Medical Center, Omaha, NE, USA

Mark G. Kortepeter, MD, MPH The Nebraska Biocontainment Unit, Department of Epidemiology, College of Public Health, University of Nebraska Medical Center, Omaha, NE, USA

Arthur M. Krasilovsky, LCSW, CEAP Faculty Staff Assistance Program, Emory University, Atlanta, GA, USA

Christopher J. Kratochvil, MD Associate Vice Chancellor for Clinical Research, University of Nebraska Medical Center, Omaha, NE, USA

Lekshmi Kumar, MD, MPH Section of Prehospital and Disaster Medicine, Department of Emergency Medicine, Emory University School of Medicine, Atlanta, GA, USA

Elena H. Kwon, DO, MPH Division of Medicine, U.S. Army Medical Research Institute of Infectious Diseases (USAMRIID), Fort Detrick, MD, USA

John J. Lowe, PhD, MS Department of Environmental and Occupational Health, College of Public Health, University of Nebraska Medical Center, Omaha, NE, USA

Syra Sikandar Madad, DHSc, MSc Director, Special Pathogens Program, Emergency Management, New York City Health + Hospitals, New York, NY, USA

John J. Maher, JD Attorney, J. Knipper and Company, Inc., Lakewood, NJ, USA

Former Director, Special Pathogens Program, New York City Health + Hospitals / Bellevue, New York, NY, USA

Jill S. Morgan, RN Serious Communicable Disease Unit, Emory University Hospital, Atlanta, GA, USA

Mallory Reimers, MSN Department of Medicine, Johns Hopkins Hospital, Baltimore, MD, USA

Anthony R. Sambol, MA Associate Director, Nebraska Public Health Laboratory, Department of Pathology and Microbiology, University of Nebraska Medical Center, Omaha, NE, USA

Lauren M. Sauer, MSc Johns Hopkins Biocontainment Unit, Johns Hopkins Hospital, Baltimore, MD, USA

Department of Emergency Medicine, Johns Hopkins University, Baltimore, MD, USA

Kathryn Shaw-Saliba, PhD, ScM Department of Emergency Medicine, Johns Hopkins University School of Medicine, Baltimore, MD, USA

Erica S. Shenoy, MD, PhD Infection Control Unit, Division of Infectious Diseases, Region 1 Ebola and Other Special Pathogens Treatment Center, Massachusetts General Hospital; Harvard Medical School, Boston, MA, USA

Karen L. Stiles, BSMT Nebraska Public Health Laboratory, Department of Pathology and Microbiology, University of Nebraska Medical Center, Omaha, NE, USA

Angela Vasa, BSN, RN, CCRN The Nebraska Biocontainment Unit, Nebraska Medicine, Omaha, NE, USA

Taylor Wilson, BS Media Relations Sr. Coordinator, Nebraska Medicine, Omaha, NE, USA

Timo Wolf, MD Associate Professor in Infectious Diseases, Head of the Isolation Unit for Highly Contagious Diseases, Department of Infectious Diseases, University Hospital, Frankfurt, Germany

1 Communicable Diseases and Emerging Pathogens: The Past, Present, and Future of High-Level Containment Care

Theodore J. Cieslak, Jocelyn J. Herstein, and Mark G. Kortepeter

Introduction

The past few decades have witnessed a number of outbreaks of communicable disease caused by novel or emerging pathogens with the potential to produce significant morbidity and mortality in humans. Although highly hazardous communicable diseases (HHCDs) such as smallpox and plague date to antiquity, the year 1969 saw a convergence of events that brought such diseases, and the pathogens that cause them, into the forefront of public consciousness. The publication, that year, of Michael Crichton's fictional work, *The Andromeda Strain*, magnified concerns initially raised by media coverage surrounding the decision to shutter the US offensive biological weapons program. The success of the Apollo 11 mission later that year and the possibility that returning astronauts might bring extraterrestrial pathogens back to earth upon their return further heightened these concerns and was partly responsible for the decision to build the first specialized units dedicated to the isolation of patients potentially harboring highly hazardous communicable pathogens [1]. These units, the Lunar Receiving Laboratory at the Johnson Manned Spaceflight Center in Houston and the "Slammer" at the US Army's Medical Research institute of Infectious Diseases (USAMRIID) at Fort Detrick MD, would usher in a new era of "high-level containment care" (HLCC) and foster a reexamination of institutional

The views expressed herein are those of the authors and do not necessarily reflect the position of the University of Nebraska or its component entities.

T. J. Cieslak (✉) · M. G. Kortepeter
The Nebraska Biocontainment Unit, Department of Epidemiology,
College of Public Health, University of Nebraska Medical Center, Omaha, NE, USA
e-mail: ted.cieslak@unmc.edu

J. J. Herstein
Department of Environmental, Agricultural & Occupational Health,
College of Public Health, University of Nebraska Medical Center,
Omaha, NE, USA

A. Hewlett, A. R. K. Murthy (eds.), *Bioemergency Planning*,
https://doi.org/10.1007/978-3-319-77032-1_1

infection control procedures. Nearly simultaneously, an emphasis on improved laboratory safety would be prompted by the 1969 discovery of the contagious and deadly viral hemorrhagic fever virus, Lassa, by researchers at Yale [2]. After a Yale technician died of laboratory-acquired Lassa fever, research activities were relocated to a new maximum-security laboratory (the predecessor of today's Biosafety-Level-4 [BSL-4] laboratories) at the Communicable Disease Center (now the Centers of Disease Control and Prevention [CDC]) in Atlanta.

USAMRIID's "Slammer" was a two-bed unit that employed engineering controls analogous to those seen in BSL-4 laboratories. Designed with the ability to isolate (care for patients infected with HHCDs) and quarantine (observation of individuals potentially exposed to these diseases), the unit was utilized for the latter role 21 times over its 40-year existence [3], but was never required to isolate a symptomatic patient, a fact which likely factored into its decommissioning in 2012.

In the meantime, partly in response to bioterrorism concerns raised by the 2001 anthrax attacks, as well as to the subsequent outbreaks of severe acute respiratory syndrome (SARS) and monkeypox, civilian HLCC units were constructed at Emory University and at the University of Nebraska. These two facilities cared for seven Ebola virus disease (EVD) patients during the 2014–2016 outbreak, while another two were cared for at the National Institutes of Health's Special Clinical Studies Unit, which had also developed HLCC capability. A tenth EVD patient was successfully managed under improvised HLCC conditions at New York's Bellevue Hospital.

While US ETCs have, as of this writing, cared for a handful of EVD victims and a single patient with Lassa fever [4], it is expected that such facilities will be ready to manage patients with a number of additional HHCDs. In this regard, we envision that four broad categories of patients might be viewed as candidates for admission to a HLCC unit (Table 1.1). We briefly discuss each of these categories, as well as the pathogens contained therein, allowing that the list of such pathogens is designed to be neither under- nor over-inclusive. In this regard, we acknowledge that some institutions may elect to care for patients in a HLCC setting even though the disease they harbor may not be included on this list, and the same patient might not necessarily be managed under HLCC conditions at another institution. Similarly, we realize that new diseases may emerge and be cared for under HLCC conditions until a certain level of confidence with their management is gained. Finally, we acknowledge that future developments in vaccinology and therapeutics may well lead to the removal of some diseases from the current list.

Patients Who Might Warrant Care in a High-Level Containment Care Unit

First, patients harboring diseases caused by pathogens that require handling under BSL-4 conditions in the laboratory would seem to be obvious candidates for clinical management under HLCC conditions. Several taxonomic families contain such highly hazardous viruses:

The orthopoxvirus, Variola (the causative agent of smallpox)
The henipaviruses, Hendra and Nipah
The filoviruses, Ebola and Marburg
The arenaviruses, which can be divided into Old World (Lassa, Lujo) and New World (Guanarito, Junin, Machupo, Sabia) agents, the latter causing Venezuelan, Argentinian, Bolivian, and Brazilian hemorrhagic fevers, respectively
The bunyavirus, Crimean-Congo hemorrhagic fever (CCHF)
The flaviviruses, Kyasanur Forest (and the closely related Alkhumra virus), Omsk hemorrhagic fever, Russian spring-summer encephalitis (as well as closely related viruses), and viruses of the tick-borne encephalitis complex (such as Absettarov, Hanzalova, Hypr, and Kumlinge)

Table 1.1 Potential candidates for management under HLCC conditions

1. Persons with diseases having the potential for person-to-person transmission whose causative agents require handling under biosafety-Level-4 conditions
Arenaviral hemorrhagic fevers
Lassa fever
Lujo hemorrhagic fever
Argentinian, Bolivian, Brazilian, Venezuelan hemorrhagic fevers
Bunyaviral hemorrhagic fevers
Crimean-Congo hemorrhagic fever
Filoviral hemorrhagic fevers
Ebola, Marburg
Henipavirus infections
Hendra
Nipah
Smallpox
2. Persons with other diseases caused by highly hazardous pathogens with the potential for person-to-person transmission
Coronavirus infections
Severe acute respiratory syndrome (SARS)
Middle East respiratory syndrome (MERS)
Influenza
Highly pathogenic avian influenza (HPAI)
Other novel and highly pathogenic influenza virus infections
Orthopoxvirus infections
Monkeypox
Pneumonic plague
Extensively drug-resistant tuberculosis (XDR-TB)
3. Persons with apparently severe diseases of unknown etiology for which optimal therapy and infection control measures are unknown
4. Persons with apparently severe diseases for which public assurance concerns might warrant management under high-level containment conditions

Of these, we advocate that patients infected with any except the flaviviruses be considered for movement to a HLCC facility. The latter do not require containment because they lack person-to-person (PTP) transmission, with naturally occurring disease being acquired solely through the bite of an arthropod vector. With the exception of variola and the henipaviruses, the remaining BSL-4 pathogens produce a clinical syndrome of viral hemorrhagic fever (VHF) in humans, and all are transmissible, to varying degrees, from PTP.

In addition to the BSL-4 pathogens, there are several other diseases that cause high morbidity and mortality, which are potentially communicable and thus might prompt management in a HLCC unit. While a lower risk to laboratorians permits the causative agents of these diseases to be handled utilizing BSL-3 or even BSL-2 precautions, in many cases, the precise nature of PTP transmission risk is unknown. We thus propose that the optimal management of patients harboring these agents take place under HLCC conditions. Included in this category are persons infected with a number of viral pathogens: the SARS or MERS coronaviruses, highly pathogenic avian influenza (HPAI) and other seemingly morbid novel influenza strains, and the orthopoxvirus, monkeypox.

In addition, while pneumonic plague, caused by the bacterium *Yersinia pestis*, is treatable with antibiotics, its high degree of contagion, almost universal lethality in the absence of prompt intervention, and narrow window of opportunity for successful postexposure treatment or prophylaxis make its management in a conventional hospital setting dangerous. Moreover, its history as a cause of frightening global pandemics and its past association with biological warfare make it a public perceptual and surety risk (see below). Finally, while most patients with pulmonary tuberculosis caused by conventional strains of *Mycobacterium tuberculosis* are readily cared for in a negative-pressure isolation room within a conventional medical facility, the recent emergence of strains of extensively drug-resistant tuberculosis (XDR-TB) provides justification of the need for high-level containment.

We allow for the certainty that new diseases will continue to emerge and that these new diseases may initially be severe yet insidious, their causative agents unidentified, and optimal means of their control unknown (*The Andromeda Strain* problem). In such circumstances, it may, on occasion, be prudent to manage and study victims in a HLCC environment. In this regard, SARS, MERS, Nipah, Hendra, and most of the VHFs could have been considered "Andromeda strains" at the time of their initial appearance.

Finally, we acknowledge that newly emerging and highly lethal diseases raise security and surety issues and that these are compounded by fears of biological warfare and terrorism. There may be circumstances, then, when it would be reasonable to manage patients in a HLCC unit in response to political, public assurance, and risk management concerns.

The Pathogens

Ebola

The 2014–2016 outbreak of Ebola virus disease (EVD) in West Africa involved at least 28,616 cases with 11,310 deaths [5]. The 25th such outbreak, larger than the previous 24 combined [6], resulted in the infection of several Western aid workers, led to their repatriation to the United States and Europe [7], and prompted the current ongoing expansion of HLCC facilities and capabilities. EVD is caused by viruses of the genus *Ebolavirus* in the family Filoviridae; the viruses derive their name from the Ebola River in the Democratic Republic of the Congo (DRC, then called Zaire), from whence the first cases were described in 1976. While the 2014–2016 outbreak was caused by the same Ebola virus (the type species, previously known as Ebola Zaire), EVD is also caused by at least three additional members of the *Ebolavirus* genus, Bundibugyo, Sudan, and Tai Forest viruses. A fifth species, Reston virus, produces fatal disease in nonhuman primates and has resulted in seroconversions among laboratory workers, but is not known to cause overt disease in humans. To date, all outbreaks of EVD have arisen in a small handful of African nations; Guinea, Liberia, and Sierra Leone accounted for the vast majority of cases during the 2014–2016 outbreak, while previous outbreaks occurred in the DRC, Congo, Gabon, Uganda, and South Sudan. While the ecology of EVD remains unclear, fruit bats likely serve as a reservoir host for the viruses [8]; outbreaks may begin when humans acquire the disease through contact with these bats or with duikers and nonhuman primates (who are also susceptible to EVD) consumed as bush meat. EVD is then transmitted from PTP through infected blood and body fluids. Given the profuse amount of vomitus and diarrhea often seen among victims, along with the high concentration of virus in those fluids, the risk of such transmission is quite high, especially among family caregivers and those involved in funeral preparations. Similarly, patients with EVD pose an extraordinary risk of nosocomial transmission through exposure to blood and other bodily fluids during medical procedures. Finally, Ebola virus persists in semen for many months after recovery, raising the possibility of sexual transmission.

Ebola has an incubation period of 2–21 days (mean 8–10 days), after which patients develop fever, headache, myalgia, and gastrointestinal symptoms. Hemorrhagic manifestations may be mild or profound, with hematemesis and hematochezia, purpura, and ecchymosis sometimes seen. Death typically occurs as a result of multi-organ failure rather than hemorrhage per se, and the mortality rate has ranged from 25% to 90%, depending on the species. Supportive care is the cornerstone of EVD management, and meticulous attention needs to be paid to hemodynamics, respiratory status, fluid balance, and electrolyte abnormalities. While no licensed antiviral therapy exists, monoclonal antibodies [9] and other experimental treatments have demonstrated great promise, and a vaccine candidate has been shown to be 100% efficacious in a postexposure vaccination trial [10]. Ebola viruses should be handled in the laboratory using BSL-4 safety measures, and the processing of clinical specimens potentially harboring these viruses should involve at least

BSL-3 precautions, as would be the case with all of the pathogens discussed in this chapter. The corpses of EVD victims are teeming with virus and pose an extreme risk to handlers and family members; they should only be handled by trained persons wearing appropriate PPE. Patients infected with Ebola were managed under HLCC conditions in multiple countries that evacuated infected expatriate healthcare and aid workers from West Africa, including Germany, Switzerland, Britain, France, Norway, Italy, Netherlands, Spain, as well as the United States. The infection of two nurses who cared for an EVD patient in a conventional hospital setting in Dallas, Texas, and the more favorable mortality rates of patients treated in HLCC conditions (18.5% compared to 37–74% in West Africa) [12] underscore the value of HLCC units in EVD management.

Marburg

Marburg virus was first described as the cause of a lethal outbreak of viral hemorrhagic fever among laboratory workers in Marburg, Germany, in 1967. The prototype member of the newly described family Filoviridae, Marburg, caused 7 deaths among the 32 victims (22% mortality rate) managed in modern German medical facilities, 6 of whom represented secondary cases attributable to PTP transmission. Only rare sporadic cases of Marburg were seen subsequently until 1998, when an outbreak occurred in Congo in which 128 of 154 known cases died (mortality rate 83%). A second large and very lethal outbreak occurred in Angola in 2004 (227 deaths among 252 victims, mortality 90%). Marburg disease typically begins, following a 3–9-day incubation period, with the onset of fever, headache, myalgia, and gastrointestinal symptoms (vomiting and diarrhea). Rash, hemorrhage, and thrombocytopenia are common, and uveitis often occurs; death results from multi-organ failure. Nosocomial transmission is well documented. Management is supportive; there are no licensed therapeutic agents available to treat Marburg hemorrhagic fever, although immune plasma has been used [11], and experimental therapies have proven efficacious in nonhuman primates [12]. Laboratories should handle Marburg virus under BSL-4 conditions. The management of patients with Marburg infection in HLCC settings has occurred in both the Netherlands [13] and Germany [14].

Lassa

Lassa virus is a member of the family *Arenaviridae* and is an important cause of viral hemorrhagic fever in West Africa. Endemic in the same region affected by the 2014–2016 EVD outbreak, Lassa causes as many as 300,000–500,000 human infections annually in Nigeria, Guinea, Liberia, Sierra Leone, and other nations in the region, where it accounts for 10–16% of all hospitalizations [15]. Seroprevalence rates in these countries range as high as 20%, attesting to the fact that many infections are mild or silent. Among patients ill enough to require hospitalization, mortality typically ranges from 15% to 20%. While most Lassa infections result from exposure (via ingestion or inhalation) to the urine and feces of *Mastomys* rats, PTP transmission is well documented, and the risk of nosocomial spread via exposure to blood and body fluids is high. Like Ebola, Lassa virus can persist in semen for several months, thus promoting sexual transmission. Symptomatic Lassa fever begins, following a 7–10-day incubation period, as a non-specific flu-like illness. Fever, myalgia, sore throat, and cough are followed by gastrointestinal symptoms and, often, by a maculopapular rash. In severe cases, manifestations of vascular leak (edema, ascites, pleural effusion) occur during the second week, as do neurologic symptoms such as seizures and coma. Overt hemorrhage occurs in only about 17% of patients [16], and death results from shock and organ failure. An elevated serum aspartate aminotransferase portends a poor prognosis, and levels above 150 IU/liter have been associated with a 55% mortality rate. It is in this group, however, that ribavirin was initially studied [17]. When administered intravenously within the first 6 days of illness, it reduced mortality to 5%. The use of ribavirin is also advocated for postexposure prophylaxis. Lassa is a BSL-4 pathogen and should be handled accordingly in the laboratory. Until the West Africa EVD outbreak, Lassa fever had been the most common VHF treated in an HLCC setting. Multiple HLCC units in Germany, Sweden, and the United Kingdom have experience managing Lassa fever patients, as does Emory University Hospital's Serious Communicable Diseases Unit, which treated a patient with Lassa in 2016. While three Lassa fever patients treated in the European facilities were medically evacuated from endemic countries, most were imported cases that were locally hospitalized and later transported to an HLCC facility [18, 19].

Lujo

Lujo virus, an Old World arenavirus closely related to Lassa, was first described in 2008 as the cause of a single outbreak of viral hemorrhagic fever involving five patients in Lusaka, Zambia, and Johannesburg, South Africa (the name, Lujo, derives from the two cities) [20]. Four of these patients died (mortality rate 80%), and there was evidence of spread to medical caregivers. Of note, the lone survivor was the only patient to receive ribavirin. No other cases have been reported as of this writing. Laboratories should handle specimens containing Lujo virus as they would those containing Lassa.

New World Arenaviruses

Guanarito, Junin, Machupo, and Sabia are members of the family *Arenaviridae* and the causative agents of Venezuelan, Argentinian, Bolivian, and Brazilian hemorrhagic fevers, respectively. The New World arenaviruses all have rodent hosts, and humans are incidentally infected, likely through exposure to aerosolized rodent excreta. Only a single case of naturally occurring (and two cases of laboratory-acquired) Sabia has been reported, and its potential for PTP and nosocomial transmission is thus unknown. Data supporting PTP transmission of Guanarito is likewise sparse. The close relationship of these agents to Junin and Machupo, however, both of which are known to be transmitted from PTP in nosocomial and other settings, prompts us to advocate for the management of patients infected with any of the four viruses under HLCC conditions. The incubation periods of these diseases are generally thought to range from 5 to 19 days (shorter in the case of parenteral exposure such as via needle stick injury), after which time patients develop fever and malaise, accompanied by headache, myalgia, vomiting, and diarrhea. Neurologic manifestations may differentiate New World arenaviral infections from other VHFs, where they are far less common. These manifestations may include hyporeflexia, tremor of the tongue and upper extremities, gait abnormalities, seizures, and coma. Leukopenia and thrombocytopenia can be profound, and signs of vascular leak, such as proteinuria and large ecchymoses, are often prominent. Mortality is approximately 15–30% in the case of Junin or Machupo [21]. As with Lassa, however, ribavirin appears quite beneficial in the treatment of New World Arenaviral infections, as does convalescent plasma [22]. Although not licensed in the United States, a Junin virus vaccine has been widely employed in Argentina and is thought to be more than 95% efficacious [23]. Limited animal data supports the possibility that it may protect against Machupo infection as well. All four of these viruses warrant the use of BSL-4 precautions in the laboratory.

Chapare, another virus closely related to the abovementioned four, was isolated from a single fatal case of hemorrhagic fever in Bolivia [24], and three fatal hemorrhagic fever cases in California were attributed to another closely related arenavirus, the Whitewater Arroyo virus [25], which is widely distributed among woodrats in the American Southwest. Whether these two viruses can be transmitted from PTP is unknown, and while many additional arenaviruses have been discovered in rodents, their role in human disease likewise remains unknown. It would seem prudent to manage patients potentially harboring such diseases under HLCC conditions when feasible and to handle their causative viruses in a BSL-4 laboratory.

Crimean-Congo Hemorrhagic Fever

Although reports of a disease consistent with Crimean-Congo hemorrhagic fever (CCHF) date to the twelfth century, the illness derives its name from a large outbreak of hemorrhagic fever in 1944–1945 among Soviet troops serving in the Crimea and a subsequent outbreak in the Belgian Congo [26]. The causative agent of CCHF is a *Nairovirus* in the family *Bunyaviridae*, the only member of this taxon requiring BSL-4 handling. Spread largely via the bite of *Hyalomma* ticks, it is endemic throughout much of this vector's range in Africa, Central Asia, the Middle East, and the Balkans [27]. Nonetheless, it also poses a significant risk of PTP transmission (the only bunyavirus apparently capable of this), with over 80 cases having occurred among healthcare personnel. On a global scale, CCHF is the most important tick-borne infection of humans, responsible for over 140 separate outbreaks since isolation of the virus in 1967. While 80% of human infections are thought to be subclinical, symptomatic CCHF presents in similar fashion to most other VHFs—following an incubation period of 1–3 days after a tick bite (or 5–6 days after exposure to the fluids of an infected person), patients typically experience the abrupt onset of fever, myalgia, and headache, often accompanied by neck stiffness and photophobia. Gastrointestinal symptoms (nausea, vomiting, diarrhea) are frequently seen, and thrombocytopenia with hemorrhagic manifestations (petechiae, ecchymoses) is often prominent. Although CCHF has a mortality rate of 10–40% in the absence of therapy, ribavirin may be beneficial in reducing mortality and in the prophylaxis of exposed contacts [28]. Despite a relatively wide geographic distribution, confirmed cases of CCHF in Western Europe are relatively rare. In 2004 and 2012, imported cases of CCHF were treated in HLCC units in France and the United Kingdom, respectively [29, 30]. Two autochthonous cases of CCHF occurred in Spain in 2016: the first patient was initially admitted to an ICU before being transported to an HLCC facility, and the second patient was a nurse who had cared for the first patient in the conventional ICU [31].

Another bunyavirus, Rift Valley fever (RVF) virus, is a relatively common cause of disease outbreaks throughout Africa and the Arabian Peninsula. Although it can cause a hemorrhagic fever syndrome in a small minority of cases, there is no evidence for PTP transmission of RVF and HLCC management is thus unnecessary.

Nipah

Nipah virus infection is caused by a paramyxovirus in the genus *Henipavirus*. It was first described in 1999 as the cause of an outbreak of respiratory illness and encephalitis in Malaysia and Singapore; during the initial Malaysian outbreak, at least 100 of 257 cases resulted in death [32], for a mortality rate of 39%. Subsequent outbreaks have been limited to Bangladesh and neighboring areas of India. While virtually all cases of Nipah infection in Malaysia and Singapore are thought to have resulted from close contact with infected pigs, PTP transmission appears to be a factor in the spread of disease during Bangladeshi outbreaks [33]. The Malaysian pigs presumably acquire the disease from *Pteropus* bats which roost in the orchards where pigs are permitted to feed on fallen fruit. In Bangladesh, a Muslim-majority nation in which pigs are seldom raised, disease appears instead to be spread via the consumption of raw date palm sap contaminated with bat excrement. Nipah has an incubation period of 5–14 days, after which time patients develop fever and headache, followed by drowsiness, confusion, and, in some cases, respiratory distress. Permanent neurologic sequelae, including personality changes and seizures, occur frequently. Treatment of Nipah is generally supportive, although ribavirin appears efficacious in vitro. Laboratories should handle Nipah virus under BSL-4 conditions.

Hendra

Like Nipah, Hendra virus infection is caused by a *Henipavirus* in the family *Paramyxoviridae*. The virus was discovered in 1994 as the cause of fatal infections among horses in Hendra, a suburb of Brisbane, Australia. Similar to the situation with Nipah, the horses appear to have contracted the disease through exposure to the secretions of infected *Pteropus* bats. Although human infection has been exceedingly rare (only seven cases have been reported as of this writing), mortality is high (4/7, 57%). Hendra appears to have an incubation period of 9–16 days, and clinical disease involves a severe respiratory illness accompanied by encephalitis. Ribavirin has in vitro activity against the virus but has not been studied in vivo. While PTP transmission of Hendra has not been documented, we feel that the similarities between this virus and Nipah, coupled with scant clinical experience, warrant extreme prudence. We thus advocate for the management of human Hendra virus infection in a HLCC setting: laboratory handling should be done under BSL-4 conditions.

The SARS Coronavirus

The severe acute respiratory syndrome (SARS) first appeared as a distinct clinical entity in the Guangdong province of China in 2002. The disease was ultimately attributed to a newly described coronavirus, a taxonomic family previously associated with the common cold. While 85% of the 8–10,000 cases associated with the 2003 epidemic occurred in China, global travel resulted in infections in 37 nations, with a mortality rate of approximately 10%. Toronto, Canada, experienced roughly 250 cases, with evidence of local PTP transmission. The disease then disappeared, and there have been no reported cases anywhere in the world since 2004. Bats appear to be the reservoir for the SARS coronavirus (SARS-CoV) and are thought to have spread the pathogen to civet cats; early human infections resulted from contact with these cats [34]. Although animal hosts may be asymptomatic, human infection with SARS-CoV results, after a 2–7-day incubation period, in an initial flu-like illness with fever, cough, sore throat, myalgia, and lethargy. This typically progresses to a severe viral pneumonia, sometimes with secondary bacterial involvement. Diarrhea and other gastrointestinal symptoms occur in a significant minority of patients. Laboratory findings often include lymphopenia, as well as elevated transaminases, lactate dehydrogenase, and creatine phosphokinase. The treatment of SARS is supportive, and BSL-3 precautions should be employed by laboratories.

During the SARS outbreak, 33 cases were imported into Western Europe, and most were treated in HLCC settings in Germany, France, Italy, Sweden, and the United Kingdom [35]. At the epicenter of the outbreak, isolation capabilities in Beijing and Singapore were exhausted quickly, and hospital complexes with HLCC capability were built for increasing numbers of SARS patients [36, 37]. In Singapore and Taiwan, insufficient space led to the temporary designation of SARS hospitals, where engineering controls were installed, contamination zones established, and PPE donning and doffing areas designated [38].

The MERS Coronavirus

The Middle East respiratory syndrome is caused by another coronavirus (MERS-CoV) closely related to SARS-CoV and was first described as the cause of an outbreak of severe and often fatal respiratory disease on the Arabian Peninsula in 2012. While autochthonous cases have been reported only in the Middle East, travel-associated cases have occurred in the United States, Western Europe, and East Asia. As of this writing, the outbreak is still ongoing, with well over 1500 cases reported; although asymptomatic infection does occur, the mortality rate of MERS is 35–40% among symptomatic patients. Person-to-person transmission occurs frequently. Following an incubation period of 2–14 days, MERS begins with non-specific flu-like symptoms and progresses, much like SARS, to a severe viral pneumonia, acute respiratory distress syndrome, and respiratory failure. Laboratory findings are similar to those seen in patients with SARS, and clinical management is likewise supportive. The World Health Organization has published comprehensive guidance for the provision of supportive care to patients with MERS [39]. MERS-CoV isolates, as well as specimens from patients suspected of having MERS, should be handled in the laboratory using BSL-3 precautions.

Highly Pathogenic Influenza Strains

Influenza is caused by a number of viruses in the family *Orthomyxoviridae*. Human infections are attributed to three genera, *influenza viruses* A, B, and C. While influenza B and C are known to cause seasonal disease in humans, only influenza A has the potential for causing devastating pandemics. This potential results from the virus's ability to exchange genes among strains, a process resulting in "antigenic shift." The most important of these genes are those coding for two viral proteins, hemagglutinin (H) and neuraminidase (N). Viral strains are characterized by these proteins, with H1N1 and H3N2 currently circulating as causes of seasonal influenza among humans. While most viruses are somewhat species specific, both human and avian strains have the ability to infect pigs; simultaneous infection of pigs risks the exchange of genetic material between human and avian strains within the porcine host. Such an exchange caused the 2009 H1N1 swine variant outbreak and, while this outbreak was milder than some feared initially, the devastating potential of novel influenza strains is best highlighted by the global 1918 Spanish flu pandemic, which is estimated to have caused 50–100 million deaths worldwide (3–5% of the world's population) [40]. Even in the absence of a pandemic, seasonal influenza causes a mean of 36,000 excess deaths annually in the United States alone, largely among the elderly. Although most patients recover from seasonal human influenza, disease caused by avian strains among poultry and aquatic birds can be devastating.

Highly pathogenic avian influenza (HPAI) H5 or H7 strains can have mortality rates of 90–100% in chickens, turkeys, and ducks. While most avian influenza viruses are not particularly infectious for humans, there is fear that a novel emerging influenza strain might combine the infectivity for humans with mortality rates seen in birds.

Seasonal influenza has an incubation period of 1–4 days, and patients may be contagious 24 h prior to the onset of symptoms, which poses a challenge to infection control efforts. Initial symptoms include fever and respiratory complaints (cough, sore throat, rhinitis), accompanied by myalgia, headache, and malaise. Primary viral and secondary bacterial pneumonias occur frequently and are often the cause of death in fatal cases. Avian influenza strains, when they do produce symptomatic disease in humans, often result in rapid progression to severe respiratory distress and respiratory (as well as other organ) failure. While supportive care is a mainstay of treatment for all forms of influenza, adamantanes (amantadine, rimantidine) and neuraminidase inhibitors (oseltamivir, zanamivir, peramivir) have been beneficial in some cases. Susceptibility to these drugs varies greatly among strains, however, and their use should be considered in view of guidelines put forth annually by the CDC and World Health Organization. Annual influenza vaccination will not protect against novel and avian strains but is useful in lowering the prevalence of seasonal influenza in the community, thereby potentially providing diminished opportunities for viral reassortment events. The sporadic occurrence of a case of influenza caused by a novel, seemingly highly pathogenic strain might merit isolation and care under HLCC conditions. In the face of a pandemic, however, HLCC bed capacity would quickly be overwhelmed, and alternative management strategies would need to be employed. Seasonal influenza virus strains, and clinical specimens harboring such strains, can be handled under BSL-2 conditions. Non-contemporary and HPAI strains warrant BSL-3 handling.

Variola (Smallpox)

Smallpox ranks as, perhaps, humanity's greatest killer. Responsible for the deaths of several hundred million people over the course of history, its eradication, the result of an intense and coordinated global effort, similarly ranks among public health's greatest achievements. Naturally occurring smallpox was last seen in Somalia in 1977, and worldwide vaccination against the disease was halted in the early 1980s. A case today would likely be the result of a laboratory accident, a bioterror attack, or a reawakening of dormant virus (e.g., from a corpse preserved in permafrost). Smallpox is caused by variola virus, a member of the *Orthopoxvirus* genus in the family *Poxviridae*. Its control was enabled by the use of a vaccine derived from vaccinia, a related, but far less pathogenic virus in the same genus. Unusual among viruses, variola is quite stable ex vivo and can survive (e.g., in crusted scab material) for decades. Smallpox is transmissible via both contact (e.g., with scabs) and droplet nuclei. Following an incubation period of 7–17 days, initial symptoms include fever, malaise, prostration, headache, and myalgia [41]. These symptoms are followed very closely by a characteristic exanthem and enanthem (lesions can be seen in the mouth and other mucosal surfaces and are present on internal organs). The rash progresses in synchronous fashion from macules to papules to vesicles to pustules to tense painful lesions said to mimic pellets embedded in the skin. The lesions are centrifugal in distribution and involve the palms and soles, differentiating them from those of chickenpox. When the disease was endemic, smallpox had a 30% mortality rate (from multisystem organ failure), and survivors were left with deep scars from these lesions.

Historically, supportive care served as the primary means of treatment for smallpox patients, although recently cidofovir [42], licensed for the treatment of cytomegalovirus retinitis, has shown promise in treating other orthopoxviruses in animal models and in immunocompromised humans. Similarly, tecovirimat has been used under an investigational new drug protocol to treat persons with complications arising from receipt of live vaccinia virus and has also demonstrated efficacy in animal *Orthopoxvirus* models [43]. As evidenced by its past success, vaccination is quite effective in preventing smallpox, and the US Strategic National Stockpile contains robust quantities of vaccinia vaccine. Administering vaccine promptly postexposure (within 4 days) may prevent or ameliorate disease, an unusual attribute among vaccines. Despite these countermeasures, an outbreak of smallpox today, occurring in an immunologically naïve population, would likely pose a significant risk of mortality, and a single case would constitute a grave public health emergency. Smallpox stores are held in only two authorized laboratories at the Centers for Disease Control and Prevention (CDC) and at the State Research Center of Virology and Technology in Koltsovo, Russia. Any handling of clinical materials potentially containing virus should only be done under tight security and BSL-4 conditions.

Monkeypox

Monkeypox is caused by an *Orthopoxvirus* closely related to variola and was only differentiated from smallpox in 1970 during efforts to eradicate the latter [44]. While its primary host appears to be macaque monkeys, it can infect humans and a number of other animals, notably rodent species. While monkeypox is endemic in the Democratic Republic of the Congo, contact with infected rodents has resulted in cases elsewhere. In 2003, an outbreak of monkeypox in the upper Midwestern United States was traced to the importation of infected Gambian giant rats. The rats transmitted the disease to prairie dogs; exposure to these rodents resulted in the infection of over 70 people [45]. In fact, fear among clinicians and refusal to care for infected patients during this outbreak [46] was one factor leading to the University of Nebraska's decision to build its HLCC unit. Human monkeypox presents a clinical picture very similar to that of smallpox, albeit with a milder course and lower mortality rate (<10%). In addition, monkeypox produces significant generalized lymphadenopathy whereas smallpox does not, perhaps indicative of more effective immune recognition [47]. It is principally for this reason—the need to rule out smallpox—that we advocate for the management of suspected monkeypox patients under HLCC conditions. Monkeypox is transmissible from PTP, and special caution is warranted until such time as smallpox is ruled out. Vaccinia vaccine administration appears protective against other orthopoxviruses, including monkeypox, and HLCC unit personnel can thus be protected through immunization. Monkeypox should be handled in the laboratory using BSL-3 precautions.

Pneumonic Plague

Few diseases conjure up images of fear and destruction as vividly as plague. The disease was first described as the cause of a great pandemic that began in Egypt in 541 AD. Known as the "Plague of Justinian," it led to the death of 50–60% of the population of Europe and is said to have sealed the fate of the Eastern Roman Empire. A second pandemic, known as the "Black Death," struck Europe in 1346 and wiped out one-third of the existing population. A third pandemic began in China in 1855 and killed at least 12 million. Plague, caused by the Gram-negative bacillus, *Yersinia pestis*, presents clinically in multiple forms, with bubonic, septicemic, and pneumonic being the most common. Bubonic plague is most often contracted by the bite of an infected flea, particularly *Xenopsylla cheopis*, the Oriental rat flea; in the United States, prairie dogs often serve as a reservoir. Pneumonic plague can be acquired primarily through exposure to infectious droplets (as might be generated by coughing or sneezing) or secondarily following the seeding of the lungs of a septicemic patient. It is this form of the disease that is readily transmissible from PTP. Pneumonic plague typically begins following an incubation period of just 2–3 days, when patients experience the abrupt onset of high fever, chills, and rapidly developing tachypnea and dyspnea. Hemoptysis, a hallmark finding in pneumonic plague, occurs within 18–24 h of symptom onset and heralds an almost universal and rapidly impending death. As a bacterial disease, plague is amenable to treatment with antibiotics; aminoglycosides (streptomycin, gentamicin), fluoroquinolones, doxycycline, and chloramphenicol are typically effective but must be started very early in the course of disease. We advocate for the management of patients with pneumonic plague under HLCC conditions due to plague's extreme infectivity, short incubation period, very rapid progression from the onset of symptoms to death, and futility of treatment once patients have become symptomatic. Preexposure and postexposure prophylaxis with oral doxycycline or ciprofloxacin may be useful in protecting healthcare workers caring for a plague victim. A licensed vaccine is currently out of production; while it provided some efficacy against bubonic plague, it was ineffective at protecting against disease acquired via inhalation. BSL-3 controls should be employed by clinical laboratories handling *Yersinia pestis* or specimens potentially containing the organism.

XDR-TB

Tuberculosis (TB) is caused by infection with the bacterium *Mycobacterium tuberculosis* (and occasionally by *M. bovis*) and has been a scourge of mankind since antiquity. Responsible for the deaths of 25% of adults in eighteenth-century Europe, the disease was brought under control with the discovery of streptomycin in 1946 and isoniazid in 1952. Most isolates of *M. tuberculosis* remain susceptible to these drugs today and to others such as rifampin, ethambutol, and pyrazinamide. Nonetheless, the recent emergence of multi-drug-resistant TB (MDR-TB) strains, defined as having resistance to both isoniazid and rifampin, is a cause for concern given the limited number of effective tuberculocidal drugs available. Even more ominous are strains of extensively drug-resistant TB (XDR-TB), defined as having resistance to isoniazid, rifampin, and fluoroquinolones, plus at least one of three "second-line" drugs (kanamycin, amikacin, and capreomycin, all of which are only effective when administered parenterally). Patients harboring such strains pose significant treatment challenges and only 30–50% achieve cure. Even in cases where treatment is ultimately successful, the period of contagion may be prolonged, and patients may require airborne isolation for many months.

One-third of the world's population has TB, although the vast majority of these persons have latent infection and are asymptomatic (and noninfectious). While tuberculous disease may involve lymph nodes, kidneys, spine, bone, and other organs, it is the pulmonary form of TB which is most common among symptomatic patients, however, and the form which poses the greatest risk of PTP transmission. Patients with symptomatic pulmonary TB typically present with chronic cough, night sweats, low-grade fever, and weight loss. Radiographic findings vary considerably, but often include hilar and paratracheal lymphadenopathy, as well as pulmonary cavitary lesions and upper lobe atelectasis or infiltrates. Most patients with pulmonary tuberculosis caused by susceptible strains are readily managed in a negative-pressure isolation room using airborne precautions. We believe, however, that disease due to MDR-TB should prompt consultation with an expert in TB management. We further advocate that disease due to XDR-TB should be considered for management in a HLCC unit; the agent, and clinical specimens potentially containing it, should be handled under BSL-3 conditions.

Discussion

The list of pathogens that might warrant care under HLCC conditions is short, and the incidence of disease caused by the majority of these pathogens, at least in developed settings, is low. This is fortunate given the very limited capacity to provide such care. While we foresee that this capacity will increase in the coming years, driven in large part by the collaborative efforts of the National Ebola Training and Education Center (NETEC), we expect that their principal benefit will derive from a reexamination and a strengthening of "conventional" infection control practices throughout the healthcare system. While some might call for a more dramatic expansion in HLCC capacity, further additions to the list of diseases managed in HLCC units, or even a return to BSL-4-like care, there is reason to proceed cautiously. HLCC, and especially BSL-4-like care, is not without disadvantages. The most obvious of these are economic. It is estimated that the average cost incurred by

US Ebola Treatment Centers in acquiring HLCC capabilities during the 2014–2016 EVD outbreak exceeded $1.19 million per hospital [48]. While some of these are one-time investments (e.g., unit construction and planning), others are ongoing operational costs, such as staff training and the maintenance of supply stocks. Moreover, the provision of care under HLCC or BSL-4-like conditions creates numerous challenges for caregivers: PPE ensembles can be awkward and clumsy and can lead to claustrophobia. They also limit the time that caregivers can spend performing direct patient care activities, and they decrement auditory and tactile sense. All of these factors risk decreasing, rather than improving, patient and provider safety. While intense training and frequent exercising assist in mitigating against these risks in existing HLCC units, they may be impractical on a larger scale.

Conversely, the management of these HHCDs outside the HLCC environment is fraught with hazard. Cases have been successfully treated in conventional hospitals when an HLCC setting was unavailable or there was a delay in diagnosis; a woman with undiagnosed Marburg virus infection was successfully managed at a community hospital in Colorado [49]. Institutional responses to such exigencies have involved modifying policies, adapting infrastructure, and relying on universal standard precautions. Such approaches, however, heighten the exposure risk to healthcare workers and can cause critical delays in treatment and laboratory testing. Documented nosocomial transmission of many of the aforementioned diseases and high infection rates among healthcare workers during the SARS and EVD outbreaks reinforce the importance of engineering controls and highly trained staff to provide safe, quality care to patients harboring highly hazardous contagious pathogens. Therefore, while these diseases may be managed safely in a conventional facility if absolutely necessary, in most cases transfer to an HLCC unit is warranted to ensure the safety of healthcare workers, other patients, and the general public.

In summary, the HLCC unit incorporates a broad range of infection control measures, engineering modifications, and personnel considerations (detailed in another chapter in this text) that differentiate it from the "conventional" negative-pressure hospital isolation ward. These serve to:

1. Protect patients by providing care in a self-contained unit staffed by selected individuals with expertise in critical care and infectious diseases
2. Protect families by removing difficult decisions about visitation
3. Protect other patients from the threat of contagion
4. Protect laboratory personnel handling specimens containing highly hazardous communicable pathogens
5. Protect the community by offering an additional level of safety, surety, and confidence
6. Protect the healthcare worker against nosocomial transmission

This latter protection is especially vital given that at least 815 cases of nosocomial Ebola occurred during the 2014–2016 West African outbreak [50], a risk to clinical personnel 21–32 times that of the general population [51].

References

1. Cieslak TJ, Kortepeter MG. A brief history of biocontainment. Curr Treat Opt Infect Dis. 2016;8:251–8.
2. Crawford DH. The invisible enemy: a natural history of viruses. Oxford: Oxford University Press; 2000.
3. Kortepeter MG, Martin JW, Rusnak JM, Cieslak TJ, Warfield KL, Anderson EL, Ranadive MV. Managing potential laboratory exposure to Ebola virus by using a patient biocontainment care unit. Emerg Infect Dis. 2008;14:881–7.
4. Balotin L. Emory hospital admits Lassa fever patient. The Emory Wheel, 15 Mar; 2016.
5. Centers for Disease Control and Prevention. 2014 Ebola outbreak in West Africa- case counts At: https://www.cdc.gov/vhf/ebola/outbreaks/2014-west-africa/case-counts.html. Accessed 13 Mar 2017.
6. Rougeron V, Feldmann H, Grard G, Becker S, Leroy EM. Ebola and Marburg haemorrhagic fever. J Clin Virol. 2015;64:111–9.
7. Uyeki TM, Mehta AK, Davey RT, et al. Clinical management of Ebola virus disease in the United States and Europe. N Engl J Med. 2016;374:636–46.
8. Leroy EM, Kumulungui B, Pourrut X, et al. Fruit bats as reservoirs of Ebola virus. Nature. 2005;438:575–6.
9. PREVAIL II Writing Group, Multi-National PREVAIL II Study Team, et al. A randomized controlled trial of ZMapp for Ebola virus infection. N Engl J Med. 2016;375:1448–56.
10. Henao-Restrepo AM, Camacho A, Longini IM, et al. Efficacy and effectiveness of an rVSV-vectored vaccine in preventing Ebola virus disease: final results from the Guinea ring vaccination, open-label, cluster-randomized trial. Lancet. 2017;389:505–18.
11. Centers for Disease Control and Prevention. Viral hemorrhagic fever: initial management of suspected and confirmed cases. MMWR. 1983;32(Suppl):S27–39.
12. Thi EP, Mire CE, Bedoya RU, et al. Marburg virus infection in nonhuman primates: therapeutic treatment by lipid-encapsulated siRNA. Sci Transl Med. 2014;6:250ra116. https://doi.org/10.1126/scitranslmed.3009706.
13. Timen A, Koopmans MP, Vossen AC, et al. Response to imported case of Marburg hemorrhagic fever, the Netherlands. Emerg Infect Dis. 2009;15:1171–5.
14. European Network of Infectious Disease Physicians. Report of the first annual meeting. Report 2005. Rome, 27–28 May 2005.
15. Ogbu O, Ajuluchukwu E, Uneke CJ. Lassa fever in West African sub-region: an overview. J Vector Borne Dis. 2007;44:1–11.
16. Brosh-Nissimov T. Lassa fever: another threat from West Africa. Dis Mil Med. 2016;2:8. https://doi.org/10.1186/s40696-016-0018-3.
17. McCormick JB, King IJ, Webb PA, et al. Lassa fever: effective therapy with ribavirin. N Engl J Med. 1986;314:20–6.
18. European Centre for Disease Prevention and Control. Lassa fever in Nigeria, Benin, Togo, Germany and USA. 23 Mar 2016, Stockholm; 2016.
19. World Health Organization. Lassa fever. http://www.who.int/csr/don/archive/disease/lassa_fever/en/. Accessed 26 Feb 2017.
20. Sewlall NH, Richards G, Duse A, et al. Clinical features and patient management of Lujo hemorrhagic fever. PLoS Negl Trop Dis. 2014;8:e3233.
21. Doyle TJ, Bryan RT, Peters CJ. Viral hemorrhagic fevers and hantavirus infections in the Americas. Infect Dis Clin N Am. 1998;12:95–110.
22. Enria D, Maiztegui JI. Antiviral treatment of Argentine hemorrhagic fever. Antivir Res. 1994;23:23–31.
23. Maiztegui JI, McKee KT, Barrera Oro JG, et al. Protective efficacy of a live attenuated vaccine against Argentine hemorrhagic fever: AHF Study Group. J Infect Dis. 1998;177:277–83.
24. Delgado S, Erickson BR, Agudo R, et al. Chapare virus, a newly discovered Arenavirus isolated from a fatal hemorrhagic fever case in Bolivia. PLoS Pathog. 2008;4:e1000047. https://doi.org/10.1371/journal.ppat.1000047.

25. Centers for Disease Control and Prevention. Fatal illness associated with a new world arenavirus—California, 1999-2000. MMWR. 2000;49:709–11.
26. Bente DA, Forrester NL, Watts DM, et al. Crimean-Congo hemorrhagic fever: history, epidemiology, pathogenesis, clinical syndrome, and genetic diversity. Antivir Res. 2013;100:159–89.
27. Shayan S, Bokaean M, Shahrivar MR, Chinikar S. Crimean-Congo hemorrhagic fever. Lab Med. 2015;46:180–9.
28. Conger NG, Paolino KM, Osborn EC, et al. Health care response to CCHF in a US soldier and nosocomial transmission to health care providers, Germany, 2009. Emerg Infect Dis. 2015;21:23–31.
29. Barr DA, Aitken C, Bell DJ, et al. First confirmed case of Crimean-Congo haemorrhagic fever in the UK. Lancet. 2013;382:1458,6736(13)61718–3.
30. Jaureguiberry S, Tattevin P, Tarantola A, et al. Imported Crimean-Congo hemorrhagic fever. J Clin Microbiol. 2005;43:4905–7.
31. European Centre for Disease Prevention and Control. Crimean–Congo haemorrhagic fever in Spain. 8 Sept 2016, Stockholm: ECDC; 2016.
32. Centers for Disease Control and Prevention. Outbreak of Hendra-like virus- Malaysia and Singapore, 1998-1999. MMWR. 1999;48:265–9.
33. Hsu VP, Hossain MJ, Parashar UD, et al. Nipah virus encephalitis reemergence, Bangladesh. Emerg Infect Dis. 2004;10:2082–7.
34. Shi Z, Hu Z. A review of studies on animal reservoirs of the SARS coronavirus. Virus Res. 2008;133:74–87.
35. Baka A, Fusco FM, Puro V, et al. A curriculum for training healthcare workers in the management of highly infectious diseases. Eur Secur. 2007;12:E5–6.
36. Kahn J. The SARS epidemic: treatment; Beijing hurries to build hospital complex for increasing number of SARS patients. New York Times, 27 Apr 2003.
37. Goh KT, Cutter J, Heng BH, et al. Epidemiology and control of SARS in Singapore. Ann Acad Med Singapore. 2006;35:301–16.
38. Fung C-P, Hsieh T-L, Tan K-H, et al. Rapid creation of a temporary isolation ward for patients with severe acute respiratory syndrome in Taiwan. Infect Control Hosp Epidemiol. 2004;25:1026–32.
39. World Health Organization. Clinical management of severe acute respiratory infections when novel coronavirus is suspected: what to do and what not to do. At: http://www.who.int/csr/disease/coronavirus_infections/InterimGuidance_ClinicalManagement_NovelCoronavirus_11Feb13u.pdf. Accessed 7 Mar 2017.
40. Taubenberger JK, Morensi DM. 1918 influenza: the mother of all pandemics. Emerg Infect Dis. 2006;12:15–22.
41. Henderson DA, Inglesby TV, Bartlett JG, et al. Smallpox as a biological weapon: medical and public health management. JAMA. 1999;281:2127–37.
42. Andrei G, Snoeck R. Cidofovir activity against poxvirus infections. Virus. 2010;2:2803–30.
43. Bolken TC, Hruby DE. Tecovirimat for smallpox infections. Drugs Today. 2010;46:109–17.
44. McCollum AM, Damon IK. Human monkeypox. Clin Infect Dis. 2014;58:260–7.
45. Centers for Disease Control and Prevention. Update: multistate outbreak of Monkeypox-Illinois, Indiana, Kansas, Missouri, Ohio, and Wisconsin, 2003. MMWR. 2003;52:642–6.
46. Reynolds G. Why were doctors afraid to treat Rebecca McLester? New York Times, 18 Apr 2004.
47. Damon IK. Status of human monkeypox: clinical disease, epidemiology, and research. Vaccine. 2011;29(suppl 4):D54–9.
48. Herstein JJ, Biddinger PD, Kraft CS, et al. Initial costs of ebola treatment centers in the United States. Emerg Infect Dis. 2016;22:350–2.
49. Centers for Disease Control and Prevention. Imported case of Marburg hemorrhagic fever—Colorado, 2008. MMWR. 2009;58:1377–81.

50. World Health Organization. Health worker infections in Guinea, Liberia, and Sierra Leone: a preliminary report, May 2015. http://www.who.int/csr/resources/publications/ebola/health-worker-infections/en/. Accessed 29 Feb 2016.
51. World Health Organization. Ebola health worker infections. http://www.who.int/features/ebola/health-care-worker/en/. Accessed 29 Feb 2016.

Designing Medical Facilities to Care for Patients with Highly Hazardous Communicable Diseases

2

Mark G. Kortepeter, Elena H. Kwon,
and Theodore J. Cieslak

Introduction

The Ebola virus disease (EVD) outbreak in West Africa from 2014 to 2016 necessitated an international response and required countries around the world to reassess their ability to manage patients with highly hazardous communicable diseases. Care facilities often serve as epicenters for the spread of such pathogens. Experience in a field setting has historically demonstrated the ability to reduce, but not eliminate nosocomial infections among healthcare providers. Despite four decades of experience managing Ebola in a field setting, an estimated 815 confirmed and suspected infections of caregivers occurred [1]. The World Health Organization estimated that care providers were 21–32 times more likely to become infected than the general population [2].

Although the establishment of containment care units preceded the EVD outbreak, the outbreak provided impetus for developed countries to make new investments in capabilities to handle patients infected with highly hazardous communicable diseases. This chapter will focus on the physical features, engineering controls,

The views expressed herein are those of the authors and do not necessarily reflect the position of the University of Nebraska or its component entities, the US Army Medical Research Institute of Infectious Diseases, the Medical Research and Materiel Command, the US Army Medical Command, the US Army, the Department of Defense, or the US Government.

M. G. Kortepeter (✉) · T. J. Cieslak
The Nebraska Biocontainment Unit, Department of Epidemiology, College of Public Health, University of Nebraska Medical Center, Omaha, NE, USA
e-mail: mark.kortepeter@unmc.edu

E. H. Kwon
Division of Medicine, U.S. Army Medical Research Institute of Infectious Diseases (USAMRIID), Fort Detrick, MD, USA

A. Hewlett, A. R. K. Murthy (eds.), *Bioemergency Planning*,
https://doi.org/10.1007/978-3-319-77032-1_2

infection control modalities, and training regimens that hospitals housing containment units have developed and implemented to adapt or design their facilities to minimize the spread of high-consequence pathogens to healthcare providers. Other medical facilities need not adapt all such features, but they can utilize some of the principles noted here for improving their own management of the unannounced patient with such an infection. This chapter will not discuss healthcare-associated infections, such as ventilator-associated pneumonia or catheter-related infections.

Background

Consideration of the need for containment care of patients with highly hazardous communicable diseases has undergone significant evolution since the discovery of Ebola virus in 1976 [3]. As we have argued previously, care of patients infected with hemorrhagic fever viruses should not be taken lightly and can be made safer for healthcare providers utilizing specialized units designed for such care [4]. The concept of containment care in the USA began in the late 1960s at the United States Army Medical Research Institute of Infectious Diseases (USAMRIID), Fort Detrick, Maryland [3]. The facility broke ground in 1967. At that time, Ebola had not yet been discovered, but other hemorrhagic fever viruses were known (Crimean-Congo hemorrhagic fever, CCHF (Crimea, 1944; Congo, 1969), Junin (Argentina, 1958), Machupo (Bolivia, 1963)). Marburg was first discovered that same year (Germany, Yugoslavia, 1967). Lassa followed (Nigeria, 1969), and Ebola emerged in two separate outbreaks in the former Zaire and Sudan in 1976 [5, 6].

In the 1960s, further impetus for the development of specialized containment care systems occurred at a time when the US program to develop offensive biological weapons was transitioned to a more defensive posture. In 1969, President Nixon officially closed the program, noting biological weapons "have massive, unpredictable, and potentially uncontrollable consequences" [7]. Along with this came the interest in management of potential casualties to reduce spread.

Other events, such as fear of extraterrestrial pathogens from the Apollo missions, fueled by the popular media [8], in addition to infections of researchers in the USA during the discovery of Lassa virus, contributed to the perceived need for containment laboratory safety and biocontainment patient care [9].

The original concept and design of the care facility at USAMRIID, affectionately known as the "slammer," was based on the model of the biosafety level 4 lab. The slammer consisted of a two-bed state-of-the-art facility and a neighboring surgical room [10, 11]. The name derived from the ominous sound produced by the closure of its heavy steel containment shower door and reflected the sense of isolation one might feel after being "locked in" the unit for a lengthy period.

"Hardwired" features that were unique to the slammer included negative pressure air handling, with HEPA-filtered intake air and double HEPA-filtered exhaust

Built-In Facility Design Features of the USAMRIID Isolation Unit (The "Slammer")

Negative pressure air handling
Intake HEPA filtration and exit double HEPA filtration in series
Decontamination shower
In-line pressurized air for use of fully encapsulating positive-pressure "space" suits
Steam sterilization of liquid waste
Pass-through autoclave
Pass-through ultraviolet light box
Dunk tank
Direct patient entry from outside the facility through a wall with hookup to portable isolation unit
On-site portable laboratory isolator
Epoxy-coated walls
Telemetry, video monitoring

air. Liquid waste drained into the laboratory sewer system that was steam sterilized prior to its release into the general waste stream. The walls were coated with epoxy paint for ease of decontamination. Caregivers could wear the "space suits" that utilized positive-pressure in-line air, analogous to those employed in the BSL-4 laboratories. The facility had its own pass-through autoclave on site, in addition to other measures to pass small objects or specimens in or out of the unit, including an ultraviolet pass box and dunk tank. Patients could also be brought directly into the unit from the outside through an external wall portal, rather than traversing the building. A specially designed shower was utilized at the end of a worker's shift to decontaminate the reusable positive-pressure suits.

The slammer was decommissioned in 2012 and converted to a training facility for new entrants into the BSL-4 laboratory. During its active period, 21 patients were observed or considered for observation after potential exposure to a variety of BSL-4 pathogens [12, 13], most of which occurred in the containment laboratories, although two of these exposures occurred in the field. Agents involved in the potential exposures included Ebola, Lassa, Machupo, and Junin viruses. The final patient (Ebola lab exposure) was admitted after a 19-year gap in 2004 [13]. None of the patients became ill or demonstrated evidence of infection.

Although USAMRIID employed the BSL-4-like slammer for quarantining exposed individuals who were asymptomatic, caregivers in field environments did not have the luxury of such extraordinary infrastructure to isolate ill patients and utilized barrier precautions (gowns, gloves, eye protection, masks, impermeable aprons), which led to significant decreases in spread of virus to caregivers [14]. Over the years, the guidelines from CDC have evolved significantly, as new information has surfaced regarding the spread of these infections [3]. Unfortunately, the 2014–2016 Ebola outbreak and some prior outbreaks [14, 15] demonstrated that

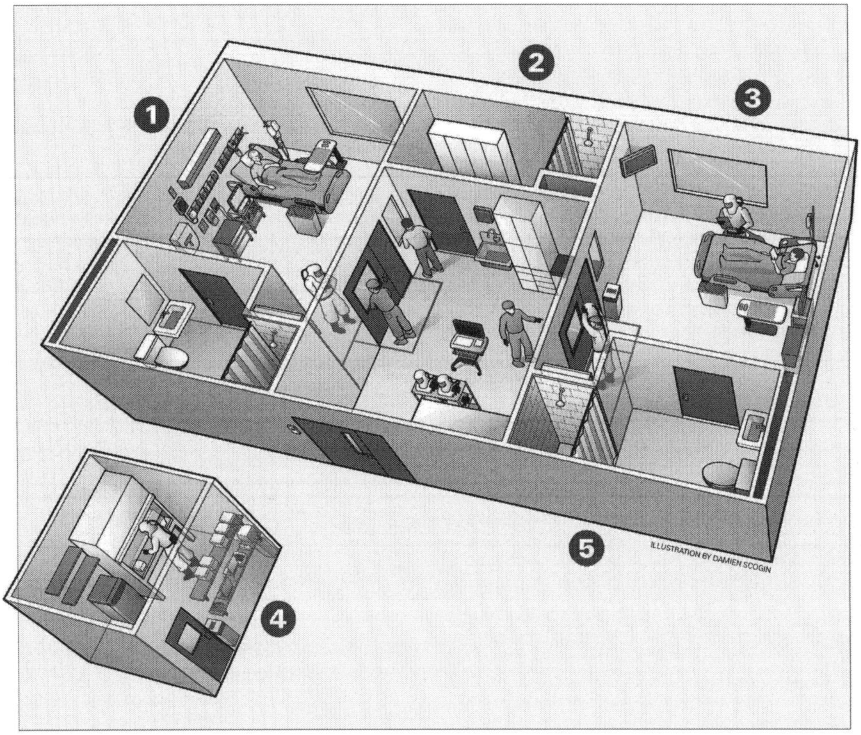

Fig. 2.1 Layout of the serious communicable disease unit at Emory University. 1 The private patient rooms resemble ICU rooms, with adjustable beds, IVs, and monitors. Every procedure a patient could need, from mechanical ventilation to hemodialysis, can be performed in the unit. 2 Medical staff who are providing direct patient care use the locker room to change into full-body protective suits and masks, which shield them from blood and bodily fluids. 3 Family members are able to speak with patients through standard glass windows in the unit; patients have access to phones and laptop computers. 4 A dedicated lab was built specifically for use with the isolation unit that has the capacity to perform blood counts, routine chemistries, blood gas measurements, urinalysis, and tests for a variety of infectious agents. 5 All liquid waste is disinfected and flushed, and disposable waste is autoclaved and incinerated. At the peak of the Ebola patients' illnesses, up to 40 bags a day of medical waste were produced. *Special Isolation Unit Schematic by Damien Scogin for Emory University is licensed under a Creative Commons Attribution 4.0 International License*

although better, the methods used in the field did not completely eliminate healthcare worker infections in those settings.

Although the military began to transition away from the slammer model, academic medical centers around the country began to develop their own specialized capabilities. Emory University opened a two-bed facility (the Serious Communicable Disease Unit, SCDU) in Atlanta in 2004 (Fig. 2.1), and the University of Nebraska Medical Center in Omaha opened a ten-bed facility in 2005 (the Nebraska Biocontainment Unit, NBU) (Fig. 2.2). The National Institute of Allergy and

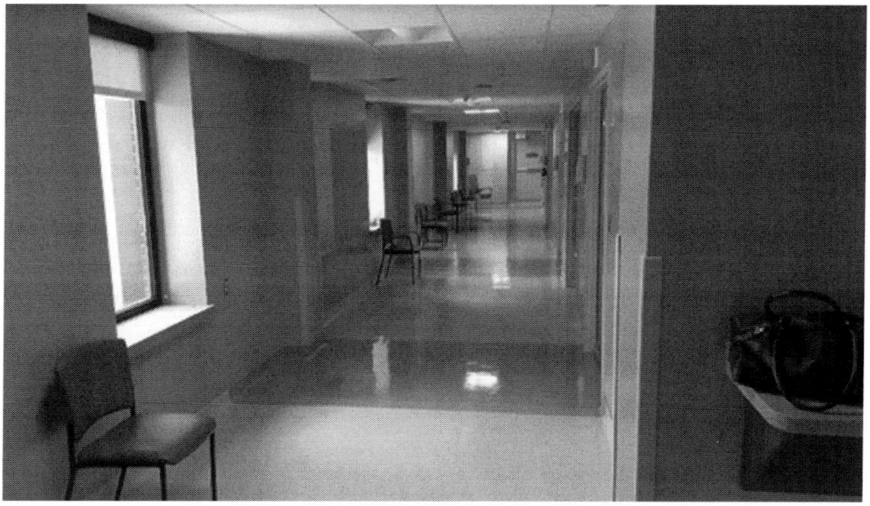

Fig. 2.2 The main patient care corridor at the University of Nebraska's Biocontainment Unit

Infectious Diseases of the NIH opened the Special Clinical Studies Unit (SCSU) in Bethesda, Maryland, in 2010.

Unlike the slammer, these facilities were outfitted inside existing medical centers, but they employed some (but not all) of the engineering features contained within the USAMRIID facility. In 2006, leaders from the three facilities in existence at the time published the first consensus guidelines for the construction, design, and employment of such units, which they dubbed "Biocontainment Patient Care Units" (BPCUs) [16]. A European Network of Infectious Diseases has published their own "framework" recommendations on design and operation of high-level containment care (HLCC) units [17].

Although care facilities don't operate under the same categorization as laboratories, as espoused in the CDC/NIH handbook on biosafety (e.g., biosafety levels 1 through 4), the USAMRIID containment unit operated under conditions that might be considered analogous to those employed in a biosafety level 4 lab (BSL-4) [18]. This level of lab safety is reserved for a handful of deadly viral pathogens for which there are no treatments or vaccines and that have the potential to infect laboratorians. In this regard, a conventional hospital room employs methods similar to a BSL-2 laboratory, while a negative pressure isolation room employs BSL-3-like controls. The HLCC units at Emory University, the University of Nebraska, and the NIH, which cared for Ebola patients during the 2014–2016 outbreak, can be viewed as BSL-3+ entities [19].

Although at one time considered to be on the fringe, some recent outbreaks have led to a reexamination of the importance of containment care facilities. The "Amerithrax" attacks of October 2001, occurring after the World Trade Center assault, and two outbreaks in 2003 added momentum, particularly as they demonstrated the risk to healthcare providers from their patients harboring lethal pathogens. The first was severe acute respiratory syndrome (SARS), a highly lethal and very contagious disease transmitted via the airborne route. The second was

Monkeypox, which arrived in the USA carried by imported Gambian giant rats. Some physicians, fearful of becoming infected, balked at treating patients infected with monkeypox [20]. The 2015 outbreak of Middle Eastern respiratory syndrome coronavirus (MERS-CoV), in Korea, led to 186 cases and significant nosocomial spread. The outbreak exposed several factors that helped facilitate the outbreak, including "late diagnosis, quarantine failure of 'super spreaders,' familial care-giving and visiting, non-disclosure by patients, poor communication by the South Korean Government, inadequate hospital infection management, and 'doctor shopping'" [21]. The concept of biocontainment became more mainstream, though, during the 2014–2016 Ebola outbreak in West Africa, as patients were brought back for care to US and European facilities [3]. The nosocomial infection of two nurses who cared for a severely ill patient in Dallas, Texas, solidified the role of biocontainment units in medicine in the USA [22].

Although there is no consensus on which patients infected with highly hazardous communicable diseases should be admitted to biocontainment units, a couple have been proposed, which are discussed in another chapter in this text. These include severe illness resulting from laboratory exposures, travel, or bioterrorism events, as well as diseases such as smallpox, monkeypox, SARS/MERS, highly pathogenic avian influenza, and those viral hemorrhagic fevers known for nosocomial spread (Ebola, Marburg, Lassa, CCHF) [16]. In addition, it makes sense for the USA to have an integrated, national network, with strategically located facilities around the country as part of an overall strategy to manage such diseases. Coordination with containment laboratory locations is reasonable, such that occupational exposures, as well as index cases of potential highly hazardous communicable diseases could be managed safely [4, 16, 23].

Design Features of Containment Units

Before a potentially infected or definitely infected patient reaches a hospital, it is useful to consider the pathway to care. For facilities that serve as a central hub or referral center from remote distances, proximity to an airfield is optimal [24]. Even when utilizing air transport, having a method for safe transport of the patient by ground to the care facility is important [25]. For suspected patients, the use of personal protective equipment (PPE) and separation of the driver component from the passenger compartment was common – this can be as simple as using layers of plastic lining the patient compartment [25, 26].

Once in the facility, having a space to evaluate suspect or ill patients at potential risk of spread is useful. During the Ebola outbreak of 2014–2016, some facilities did this in their intensive care units rather than in the emergency department. Planning in advance is key when considering transport of a patient within a facility. It is important to designate preplanned entry points and transport routes within the facility (preferably shorter distances or more direct routes to minimize contamination risk en route), including predesignated elevators and prearranged security to cordon off those routes during patient transport [27]. In some instances, individual patient isolation systems were used during ambulance or intra-facility transport [24].

The biocontainment units at Emory University, University of Nebraska, and the NIH cared for nine Ebola-infected patients during the 2014–2016 outbreak without any spread to caregivers, thus confirming the ability to care for these patients safely in a developed setting. One patient was also cared for at the New York University-Bellevue Hospital in New York City, demonstrating that with adequate precautions and infection control measures, other hospitals may be able to do this safely; however, the nosocomial transmission experience of the Dallas Presbyterian hospital also demonstrates that the virus is unforgiving and that unprepared facilities could have significant challenges [22]. There is no room for error [4].

The Europeans and Americans have come up with recommendations on the types of design features that should be included in biocontainment units [16, 17]. These include designation of "cold, warm, and hot" or "clean" and "contaminated" areas in the units, adopted from nomenclature used in containment labs. These demarcations help guide access by individuals with different skill sets and the appropriate PPE in different locations in the units. Having the appropriate space for storage, donning and doffing of equipment must also be considered. A consensus group in the USA, which included representatives from biocontainment units and containment laboratories, also developed consensus guidelines on recommended features of facilities that care for accidental exposures in labs to biosafety level-3 and level-4 agents [23].

The three currently designated national facilities have dedicated units that are physically separated from other patient care areas. These facilities are of varying sizes: the Nebraska unit has ten beds in five rooms; the NIH unit has four rooms, with seven beds; and the Emory unit has two rooms, each with single beds [28]. Numbers of beds do not adequately represent the number of patients that could be cared for. Logistically, more patients with a respiratory disease (SARS, MERS-CoV) might be able to be cared for, than EVD patients, depending on their disease acuity.

The personnel burden to care for a single patient with Ebola in the containment units numbered in the dozens, making caring for more than one or two ill patients extremely challenging. In order to minimize the number of individuals who need to enter the "hot" patient care area, units have set up video monitoring equipment and use of electronic medical record charting. Video monitoring also can be useful for communication with the patient by medical staff or communication between patients and family members, who are not allowed to enter the unit [29].

Air handling and directional airflow with sequential pressure differentials is a major feature, with units' air handling separate from the rest of the medical facility, with HEPA filtration upon exit, and with negative pressure airflow. Backup generators are used in case of power outage. Other features include secured access, the ability to control and monitor entry and egress from the facility, and dunk tanks for passing specimens out of the containment unit. Other options that have been used include pass-through autoclaves and ultraviolet light boxes. Having an occupational health program to monitor anyone entering the facility is an important adjunct. Units have used sealed floors and walls for ease of decontamination after patient discharge, although the housekeeping is frequently done by those who work on the unit, rather than ancillary personnel, who are kept to a minimum.

Within the care areas, having all the necessary life-support equipment for patient care is important to minimize the movement of equipment such as plain film radiology, ultrasound, dialysis, and ventilator equipment in and out of the care area. Other design features include hands-free or self-closing doors and ready access to handwashing facilities (hands-free, if possible).

Ready access to laboratory testing is key to minimize sending potentially contaminated patient samples to the main hospital laboratory. Units have used a combination of on-site testing with "point of care" assays for routine labs. In addition, the three units that cared for Ebola patients in the USA have established their own on-site labs.

Waste handling turned out to be one of the major unexpected challenges during the Ebola outbreak [30–32]. In the old "slammer" model, this was not an issue, since caregivers in fully encapsulated "space" suits passed through a decontamination shower when leaving the unit and suits were reused. This minimized the need for autoclaving. With the use of disposable suits, PAPR hoods, gloves, face shields, aprons, and booties, the amount of PPE waste was enormous. Patient waste was another unexpected challenge, due to the profound volume of emesis, diarrhea, and contamination of clothing and linens. On a given day, up to 40 bags of medical waste could be generated for a sick patient [33]. Units adapted by putting in pass-through autoclaves (usually more than one for redundancy to allow for maintenance of one while remaining operational). Areas need adequate space for storage of solid waste, in case the autoclaves malfunction. Specific validation of autoclave protocols, along with proper waste packaging, may also be needed, to ensure effective decontamination, depending on the agent in question [34]. Handling of waste must take into consideration for textiles (linens, pillows, mattresses, and privacy curtains) in addition to solid waste. Liquid waste handling was also a challenge [30–32]. Most facilities don't have the luxury of a steam sterilization plant on-site, as the slammer facility did. They used expedient measures such as pouring Micro-Chem Plus (Emory SCDU) or "Ecolab neutral disinfectant cleaner" (NBU) into the toilets, with an appropriate contact time, prior to releasing to the general sewage stream. Placing a cover over the toilet prior to flushing limits the potential for droplet spread. Different health departments may have local requirements for such handling.

When a patient is discharged or succumbs to the disease, it is useful to have procedures in place for decontaminating the facility and for proper care and transport of the deceased. In the NBU, when one patient succumbed to Ebola infection, visitation by the family was facilitated by a video link. Afterward, the remains were wrapped in bedsheets and placed in a biosafety level 4 containment bag. The bag was then transferred into an 18-mil thick leakproof laminated vinyl bag, followed by a second one. After a patient discharge, the room was left undisturbed for 48 h (this has the effect of allowing most pathogens to succumb to desiccation), followed by manual disinfection and ultraviolet germicidal irradiation using four UV light generators. Floors were mopped twice with a hospital disinfectant, and medical equipment was manually disinfected [32].

The Nebraska Biocontainment Unit provided a description of lessons learned from the 2014–2016 Ebola outbreak that might benefit others [26]. It was useful to have dedicated space for staff changing and storage of PPE. Patient rooms had seamless surfaces for ease of decontamination. The unit was located in a secured area separate from the rest of the hospital. This provides reassurance to the patients elsewhere in the facility and the public at large. Unit entrances and exits were monitored. Having a well-trained, competent, and interdisciplinary team of providers, appropriate protocols for PPE donning and doffing and specimen and waste handling were useful. Including laboratorians on the team, and limiting labs to point of care testing in the patient room or a biosafety cabinet in close proximity to patient, is also useful.

In response to the Ebola outbreak and being cognizant of the need for better national preparedness, Europe has developed its own network of isolation facilities within the European Network for Highly Infectious Diseases (EuroNHID) project. In the USA, the CDC recommended a three-tiered system for evaluation and management of patients with suspected or confirmed Ebola infection. While the system was initially created in response to the 2014–2016 Ebola outbreak, it is expected that participating facilities will be able to manage patients potentially infected with a number of other high-consequence pathogens, such as those noted in an accompanying chapter in this text.

These three tiers include "frontline" facilities, Ebola assessment hospitals, and Ebola treatment centers [35]. Dovetailed with this recommendation, the US Department of Health and Human Services has designated one facility in each of ten Federal Emergency Management Agency (FEMA) regions around the USA as regional "Ebola and Other Special Pathogen Treatment Centers" [36]. Three of those facilities, Emory University, University of Nebraska, and Bellevue Hospital, have been designated as national treatment centers. These three centers have joined in a consortium called the National Ebola Training and Education Center (NETEC), which trains caregivers on PPE and provides education site assessments of hospitals. Other facilities around the country have met certain criteria to serve as Ebola treatment centers, which include the following elements: operational coordination, staffing and training, clinical competency, PPE, policies and procedures for healthcare worker safety, laboratory safe work practices, private care rooms with designating donning/doffing spaces, inter-facility transportation plans, and waste management [36]. Even among these facilities, design features appear to be vastly different. For example, 94% of them have their isolation unit within the main hospital building, 43% have separate wards, 51% have separate rooms within another ward, 3 (6%) are stand alone, and 70% have separate air handling systems, and of the 24 units inside other wards, 14 (58%) have independent air handling systems. Twenty-three of those twenty-four (96%) have a physical barrier separating the isolation units. Only 10 of the 47 ETCs that responded to a survey on capabilities had all of the following: negative pressure isolation, an anteroom, on-site sterilization with autoclaves, and HEPA filtration. Some of the major limitations of these units include bed capacity and the need for dedicated, multidisciplinary staff [36].

Adapting Design Features for More General Use

Even with appropriate isolation precautions, nosocomial transmission of infectious diseases, such as tuberculosis, measles, SARS, smallpox, and other diseases, may occur, so it is reasonable for all facilities to be prepared [16, 37]. While we recognize the advantages of caring for certain highly hazardous communicable diseases within biocontainment units, we note that a principle benefit of NETEC efforts will derive from a reexamination and a strengthening of "conventional" infection control practices throughout the healthcare system.

All hospitals need not attempt to build biocontainment units, but hospitals, in general, should have some kind of plan to prepare for the possibility that a patient with a highly hazardous communicable disease could arrive at their facility unexpectedly. In this vein, some of the features embraced by biocontainment units might be adopted by other facilities. One key feature is early identification and triage of such patients at the places where they are most likely to present for care – in the emergency room or acute care and primary care clinics. Assessments of patient flow within a facility and potential contact points between patients and caregivers, family members, and other patients are a critical part of risk assessment. Having protocols in place to query patients about recent travel, ill contacts, or respiratory illness may be beneficial in those areas. Preparation for all comers and ensuring procedures for evaluation are as "idiot proof" as possible is key, because variable adherence is a huge challenge. Therefore, staff members potentially involved will require regular reinforcement with practice, testing, and management.

Some simple design features should be achievable for most facilities, such as designating a location separate from other patient care areas, but still readily accessible by staff, as a holding or triage area as well as an appropriate treatment area [27]. This need not be a locked or secured ward, as has been utilized in the containment units – simply a separate designated area. This would include some neighboring space for staff changing, storage space for PPE, and possibly an on-site shower [24, 38]. Positioning the isolation area a short distance from the entry point into the facility and laboratory assets, thus reducing the length of passage through the facility of a potentially communicable patient or potentially contaminated laboratory samples, should reduce potential risk to others [26]. The patient room should be equipped with surfaces that are easy to wipe down for disinfection, and designated equipment should be selected for easy decontamination. Having a room capable of negative pressure air handling, independent from the hospital's primary air handling system, with HEPA-filtered exhaust, is a plus. Other general features include easy access to hand washing stations and PPE [35].

Lenaghan and Schwedhelm provide a nice summary of the stages that the Nebraska Biocontainment Unit went through to bring the unit from a concept to fully operational [39]. This included a design phase with input from multiple sources, where issues such as air handling systems, the sewer system, transport of linens, waste, safety, security, mortuary, and emergency medical systems were discussed. Features planned for included access and egress of patients, materials, and supplies as well as patient transport. The unit went to great lengths to vet the appropriate staff and provide adequate orientation. Ensuring individuals interested in participating embrace the culture of safety and are willing to work in a team environment is very important. In addition, time spent in PPE can be physically demanding, and working in such an environment is stressful, so individuals should be screened for a minimum level of fitness – both physical and also psychological. The second phase included addition of video monitoring capability and text messaging. Unit leadership empowered all team members to be equally accountable for safety. Unit personnel engaged in regular drills and debriefs, and larger drills brought in organizations outside the hospital facility, such as the regional airport, the local US Air Force base, and the state health department. Unit activation occurred in advance of the first patient arriving in September 2014.

Risi et al. [40] provide a summary of how a facility might be upgraded using existing space. Key aspects emphasized included "redundant engineering of safety features, strict administrative oversight, biosecurity measures, and extensive training." Upgrades included access control, three stand-alone rooms (with bathroom and shower), an anteroom for each, directional airflow, a dedicated exhaust system with HEPA filtration, construction of seamless surfaces for topical disinfection, capability for full range of ICU care, and a separate autoclave. When not needed for the care of patients with highly hazardous communicable diseases, the rooms operate as conventional ICU beds.

Although this chapter is focused on facility design, design elements are just one important aspect for reducing the spread of infections in a healthcare setting. It is worth noting that despite a facility's layout or the type of PPE used, limiting the spread of infection relies on people. It starts with having a workplace culture and climate of safety [41]. Infrastructure is of little utility without appropriate policies and procedures for safety [35]. This comes from the top down. It also includes appropriate redundancies, appropriate levels of staffing, recurrent training and observation of procedures, and having the right, interested caregivers, who are willing to work within a team and follow procedures. Any planning is only as strong as the weakest link. Gershon found six foundational elements for a successful climate of safety [42]. These include senior management support, absence of workplace barriers to safe work practices, worksite cleanliness/orderliness, good staff communication and minimal conflict, frequent training and safety-related feedback by supervisors, and PPE availability and engineering controls.

Multiple potential barriers exist to implementing infection control guidelines in a crisis, including lack of imperative or precise wording, lack of easily identifiable instructions, lack of concrete performance targets, and lack of timely and adequate guidance on PPE or other aspects [43]. As noted by Brett-Major et al., care must be deliberate, every procedure must be practiced and follow risk/benefit, and anyone on the team can and should call a safety stop if unsafe practices are observed [44]. Training, repeatedly reinforced, is at least as important, if not more important than the physical infrastructure and the specific PPE utilized. Finally, significant communications among all aspects of care, early and often, are tantamount to appropriate preparedness and care when needed [29].

In summary, we have discussed different design features that have been incorporated in specialized biocontainment units at strategic locations around the country. Not every hospital can develop such complex infrastructure, but hospitals should decide which aspects they would like to adopt to minimize the risk of spread of hazardous pathogens to their healthcare staff. More importantly, ensuring individuals have adequate training, repeatedly reinforced, in basic infection control practices, can go a long way to reducing healthcare provider risk of spread for routine as well as exotic diseases.

References

1. World Health Organization. Health worker Ebola infections in Guinea, Liberia and Sierra Leone, Preliminary report. Found at http://www.who.int/csr/resources/publications/ebola/health-worker-infections/en/. 20 Jan 2017.
2. World Health Organization. Ebola health worker infections. Found at http://www.who.int/features/ebola/health-care-worker/en/ 24 Apr 2017.
3. Kortepeter MG, Kwon EH, Hewlett AL, Smith PW, Cieslak TJ. Containment care units for managing patients with highly hazardous infectious diseases: a concept whose time has come. J Infect Dis. 2016;214:S137–41.
4. Kortepeter MG, Smith PW, Hewlett AL, Cieslak TJ. Caring for patients with Ebola: a challenge in any care facility. Ann Int Med. 2015;162:68–9.
5. World Health Organizations. Ebola haemorrhagic fever in Zaire, 1976. Bull World Health Organ. 1978;56:271–93.
6. World Health Organization. Ebola haemorrhagic fever in Sudan, 1976. Report of a WHO/International Study Team. Bull World Health Organ. 1978;56:247–70.
7. Tucker JB, Mahan ER. President Nixon's decision to renounce the U.S. offensive biological weapons program. Washington, DC: National Defense University Press; 2009.
8. Crichton M. The Andromeda strain. New York: Centesis Corporation; 1969.
9. Crawford DH. The invisible enemy: a natural history of viruses. Oxford: Oxford University Press; 2000.
10. Covert NM. Cutting edge: a history of Fort Detrick, Maryland. 3rd ed. Fort Detrick: Public Affairs Office, Headquarters U.S. Army Garrison; 1997. p. 79.
11. Hill EE, McKee KT. Isolation and biocontainment of patients with highly hazardous infectious diseases. J Army Medical Dept. 1991;PB8–91-1/2:10–4.
12. Cieslak TJ, Christopher GW, Eitzen EM. The "slammer": isolation and biocontainment of patients exposed to biosafety level 4 pathogens. Clin Infect Dis. 1999;29:1083.
13. Kortepeter MG, Martin JW, Rusnak JM, et al. Managing potential laboratory exposure to Ebola virus by using a patient biocontainment care unit. Emerg Infect Dis. 2008;14:881–7.
14. Pigott DC. Hemorrhagic fever viruses. Crit Care Clin. 2005;21:765–83.
15. Borchert M, Mutyaba I, Van Kerkhove MD, Lutwama J, et al. Ebola haemorrhagic fever outbreak in Masindi District, Uganda: outbreak description and lessons learned. BMC Infect Dis. 2011;11:357.
16. Smith PW, Anderson AO, Christopher GW, et al. Designing a biocontainment unit to care for patients with serious communicable diseases: a consensus statement. Biosecur Bioterror. 2006;4:351–65.
17. Banniser B, Vincenzo P, Fusco FM, Heptonstall J, Ippolito G, EUNID Working Group. Framework for the design and operation of high-level isolation units: consensus of the European Network of Infectious Diseases. Lancet Infect Dis. 2009;9:45–56.
18. U.S. Department of Health and Human Services. Biosafety in microbiological and biomedical laboratories. 5th ed; 2009. Atlanta: HHS Publication No. (CDC) 21–1112.

19. Cieslak TJ, Kortepeter MG. A brief history of biocontainment. Curr Treat Opt Infect Dis. 2016;8:251–8.
20. Reynolds G. Why were doctors afraid to treat Rebecca McLester? New York Times, 18 Apr 2004.
21. Kim KH, Tandi TE, Choi JW, Moon JM, Kim MS. Middle East respiratory syndrome coronavirus (MERS-CoV) outbreak in South Korea, 2015: epidemiology, characteristics and public health implications. J Hosp Infect. 2017;95:207–13.
22. Poor planning, communication lead to missteps in care of Ebola patient. ED Manag. 2015;27(11):121–6.
23. Jahrling P, Rodak C, Bray M, Davey RT. Triage and management of accidental laboratory exposures to biosafety level-3 and -4 agents. Biosecur Bioterror Biodef Strat Pract Sci. 2009;7:135–43.
24. Beam EL, Boulter KC, Freihaut F, Schwedhelm S, Smith PW. The Nebraska experience in biocontainment patient care. Pub Health Nurs. 2010;27:140–6.
25. Lowe JJ, Jelden KC, Schenarts PJ, Rupp LE Jr, Hawes KJ, Tysor BN, Swansiger RG, Schwedhelm SS, Smith PW, Gibbs SG. Considerations for safe EMS transport of patients infected with Ebola virus. Prehosp Emerg Care. 2015;19:179–83.
26. Hewlett AL, Varkey JB, Smith PW, Ribner BS. Ebola virus disease: preparedness and infection control lessons learned from two biocontainment units. Curr Opin-Infect Dis. 2015;28:343–8.
27. Wadman MC, Schwedhelm SS, Watson S, Swanhorst J, Gibbs SG, Lowe JJ, Iwen PC, Hayes AK, Needham S, Johnson DW, Kalin DJ, Zeger WG, Muelleman RL. Emergency department processes for the evaluation and management of persons under investigation for Ebola virus disease. Ann Emerg Med. 2015;66:306–14.
28. Courage KH. Inside the 4 U.S. biocontainment hospitals that are stopping Ebola. Scientific Am 2014. Found at https://www.scientificamerican.com/article/inside-the-4-u-s-biocontainment-hospitals-that-are-stopping-ebola-video/. 24 Mar 2017.
29. Johnson DW, Sullivan JN, Piquette CA, Hewlett AL, Bailey KL, Smith PW, Kalil AC, Lisco SJ. Lessons learned: critical care management of patients with Ebola in the United States. Crit Care Med. 2015;43:1157–64.
30. Lowe JJ, Gibbs SG, Schwedhelm SS, Nguyen J, Smith PW. Nebraska biocontainment unit perspective on disposal of Ebola medical waste. Am J Infect Control. 2014;42:1256–7.
31. Lowe JJ, Olinger PL, Gibbs SG, Rengarajan K, Beam EL, Boulter KC, Schwedhelm MM, Hayes AK, Kratochvil CJ, Vanairsdale S, Frislie B, Lewis J, Hewlett AL, Smith PW, Gartland B, Ribner BS. Environmental infection control considerations for Ebola. Am J Infect Control. 2015;43:47–9.
32. Jelden KC, Gibbs SG, Smith PW, Schwedhelm MM, Iwen PC, Beam EL, Hayes AK, Narion N, Kratochvil CJ, Boulter KC, Hewlett AL, Lowe JJ. Nebraska biocontainment unit patient discharge and environmental decontamination after Ebola care. Am J Infect Control. 2015;43:203–5.
33. Leligdowicz A, Fischer WA, Uyeki TM, Fletcher TE, Adhikari NKJ, Portella G, et al. Ebola virus disease and critical illness. Crit Care. 2016;20:217–31.
34. Garibaldi BT, Reimers M, Ernst N, Bova G, Nowakowski E, Bukowski J, Ellis BC, Smith C, Sauer L, Dionne K, Carroll KC, Maragakis LL, Parrish NM. Validation of autoclave protocols for the successful decontamination of Category A medical waste generated from the care of patients with serious communicable disease. J Clin Micro. 2017;55:545–51.
35. Centers for Disease Control. Interim guidance for U.S. hospital preparedness for patients under investigation (PUIs) or with confirmed Ebola Virus Disease (EVD): a framework for a tiered approach. Found at https://www.cdc.gov/vhf/ebola/healthcare-us/preparing/hospitals.html. 20 Jan 2017.
36. Herstein JJ, Biddinger PD, Kraft CS, Saiman L, Gibbs SG, Le AB, Smith PW, Hewlett AL, Lowe JJ. Current capabilities and capacity of Ebola treatment centers in the United States. Infect Cont Hosp Epi. 2016;37:313–8.
37. Siegel JD, Rhinehar E, Jackson M, Chiarrello L, the Healthcare Infection Control Practices Advisory Committee. 2007 Guideline for isolation precautions: preventing transmission of

infectious agents in healthcare settings. Found at https://www.cdc.gov/hicpac/pdf/isolation/isolation2007.pdf. Jan 2017.
38. Beam EL, Schwedhelm SS, Boulter K, Kratochvil C, Low J, Hewlett A, Gibbs SG, Smith PW. Personal protective equipment processes and rationale for the Nebrask biocontainment unit during the 2014 activations for Ebola virus disease. Am J Infect Control. 2016;44:340–2.
39. Lenaghan PA, Schwedhelm M. Nebraska biocontainment unit design and operations. J Nurs Admin. 2015;45:298–301.
40. Risi GF, Bloom ME, Hoe NP, Arminio T, Carlson P, Powers T, Feldmann H, Wilson D. Preparing a community hospital to manage work-related exposures to infectious agents in biosafety level 3 and 4 laboratories. Emerg Infect Dis. 2010;16:373–8.
41. Moore D, Gamage B, Bryce E, Copes R, Yassi A. Protecting health care workers from SARS and other respiratory pathogens: organizational and individual factors that affect adherence to infection control guidelines. Am J Infect Control. 2005;33:88–96.
42. Gershon RR, Karkashian CD, Grosch JW, Murphy LR, Escamilla-Cejudo A, Flanagan PA, et al. Hospital safety climate and its relationship with safe work practices and workplace exposure incidents. Am J Infect Control. 2000;28:211–21.
43. Timen A, Hulscher MEJL, Rust L, van Steenbergen JE, Akkermans RP, Grol RPTM, van der Meer JWM. Barriers to implementing infection prevention and control guidelines during crises: experiences of health care professionals. Am J Infect Control. 2010;38:726–33.
44. Brett-Major DM, Jacob ST, Jacquerioz FA, Risi GF, Fischer WA 2nd, Kato Y, Houlihan CF, Crozier I, Bosa HK, Lawler JV, Adachi T, Hurley SK, Berry LE, Carlson JC, Button TC, McLellan SL, Shea BJ, Kuniyoshi GG, Ferri M, Murthy SG, Petrosillo N, Lamontagne F, Porembka DT, Schieffelin JS, Rubinson L, O'Dempsey T, Donovan SM, Bausch DG, Fowler RA, Fletcher TE. Being ready to treat Ebola virus disease patients. Am J Trop Med Hyg. 2015;92:233–7.

Administrative Considerations When Preparing for Bioemergencies

3

John J. Maher, Syra Sikandar Madad, and Nicholas V. Cagliuso Sr.

Introduction

The healthcare delivery system will always be on the frontline in response to bioemergencies. From naturally occurring events such as influenza to intentional acts such as the release of anthrax, adequate preparation for these incidents requires a unified administrative response across healthcare's myriad of entry points. Central to this is ensuring that the healthcare system maintains a knowledge of key concepts and allocation of resources necessary to maintain employee safety while ensuring that patients receive safe, effective, and efficient care. Since responding to bioemergencies requires a level of internal and external coordination that generally exceeds day-to-day healthcare system operations, healthcare entities typically rely on an emergency management approach to marry resources in real time to manage these events. This chapter applies a general emergency management approach to bioemergencies, highlights anticipated costs (and the means to track them), and considers the focal points of training staff to safely screen and isolate patients in the unclear regulatory and accreditation environment in which bioemergencies occur.

J. J. Maher
J. Knipper and Company, Inc., Lakewood, NJ, USA

Special Pathogens Program, New York City Health + Hospitals / Bellevue, New York, NY, USA

S. S. Madad
Special Pathogens Program, Emergency Management, New York City Health + Hospitals, New York, NY, USA

N. V. Cagliuso Sr. (✉)
Emergency Management, New York City Health + Hospitals, New York, NY, USA
e-mail: Nicholas.Cagliuso@nychhc.org

A. Hewlett, A. R. K. Murthy (eds.), *Bioemergency Planning*,
https://doi.org/10.1007/978-3-319-77032-1_3

Emergency Management

Implicit to successfully managing the preparation for and response to bioemergencies is employing an emergency management approach. An all-hazards emergency management paradigm addresses the full spectrum of incidents that can negatively impact the environment of care, whether they occur naturally, technologically, or intentionally. This also offers a modular and scalable means that provides healthcare administrators with the flexibility to do so safely and effectively. There are two prevailing themes when healthcare administrators consider preparing for bioemergencies: (i) bioemergencies significantly strain the day-to-day operations of a healthcare system and (ii) facilities must prepare for worst-case scenarios and scale their responses to fit the particular bioemergency at hand. A chronic challenge in healthcare emergency management is melding its principles into daily operations [1]. Too often, administrators view such efforts as binary; that is, falsely believing it can be quickly turned on or off as necessary. In truth, doing so is both highly ineffective and, at worst, unsafe. Instead, the most effective approach is to scale emergency management efforts to reflect a measured approach to situational awareness, wherein the healthcare system is constantly monitoring its internal status and the status of potential threats. To that end, when responding to bioemergencies, facilities should rely on their hospital incident command system (HICS) to ensure sustainment of their core functions of providing contemporaneous care of all other patients within their facilities. Relying on a HICS-based response to a bioemergency requires meticulous preparation, in the form of incident response guides (IRG) with corresponding job action sheets (JAS). Since all bioemergencies will be unique, the emergency management approach, relying on detailed (yet flexible) checklists and standard operating procedures, offers a healthcare system the best means to safely and effectively respond to these challenging events.

From a preparedness standpoint, since the number of bioemergency scenarios is infinite, the best approach to preparing to respond to bioemergencies is to prepare for the most likely worst-case scenario. For example, when preparing for special pathogens, such as Ebola, healthcare systems should build a robust response system and scale those responses to infectious diseases with less dire consequences. This principle is based on an all-hazards approach to emergency events, enabling the efficient allocation of scarce clinical, operational, and financial resources.

Another benefit of preparing for bioemergencies through an emergency management lens is the method of exercising and generating improvement plans to emphasize strengths and enable the correction of weaknesses. Once a healthcare system has established a HICS-based approach to bioemergencies, each facility should then conduct tabletop and full-scale exercises to test their approaches. Homeland Security Exercise Evaluation Program (HSEEP) compliant [2] after action reports and improvement plans will identify strengths and gaps and provide a timeline to addressing gaps and the accountability for doing so.

Leadership Team

Leadership is at the core of administrative considerations when preparing for bioemergencies. The ability to set direction – and adhere to it – especially during times of crisis often decides incident outcomes and is the responsibility of healthcare leadership day in and day out. Far too frequently, leadership, citing competing priorities, does not view emergency management efforts as mission-critical functions. However, incident after incident teach us that strong support from the highest levels of the organization lead to strong emergency management programs.

As such the healthcare organization's board, chief executive officer, chief operating officer, chief medical officer, and chief financial officer must set a tone of organizational resilience as daily operating requirement akin to other maxims such as "do no harm." Gone are the days when delegating emergency management projects as a part-time function to already overburdened staff suffices. On the contrary, today's healthcare delivery entities must, for good practices and to comply with myriad regulatory and accreditation standards, actively engage all levels of the organization in emergency management. From understanding how emergency management supports the organizational vision and mission to its application in the most routine tasks, such as hand hygiene efforts, leadership has the moral obligation to ensure that all are engaged and prepared.

Specific to bioemergencies, in addition to the entity's c-suite guiding efforts, subject matter experts such as infectious disease practitioners must have a clear voice and decision-influencing HICS roles to ensure that the nuances of these incidents drive actions.

Public Partnerships

While public partnerships are always important when hospitals prepare for and respond to large-scale emergencies, a HICS-based approach to bioemergencies requires a particular focus of marrying public resources to ensure a unified response. The national and local preparations and successful responses to Ebola were a case study of the importance of public partnerships when responding to special pathogens.

Preparing for bioemergencies may best be approached by working from the federal level down to the local levels of public response. A healthcare system should first seek guidance from ASPR and the CDC and ensure open lines of communications with their regional representatives. This will ensure that the system's response adheres to federal regulations (e.g., DOT transport requirements) and will ensure that particular responses, which require national coordination (e.g., shipping lab specimens), are expedited due to existing relationships and vetted procedures. Once a healthcare system has conformed to the national framework for responding to bioemergencies, the system should look toward regional resources (i.e., regional Ebola and special pathogen treatment centers and the National Ebola Training and Education Center) to borrow or improve upon best practices.

While consulting federal and regional resources is a good place to start, each healthcare system's HICS response must consider the local intricacies of their response – most importantly, coordinating with state (and sometimes city) health departments. When dealing with bioemergencies, even simple daily occurrences in a healthcare system can be stalled by a myriad of conflicting regulations and legal requirements. For example, transferring a patient from one healthcare facility to another will require meticulous planning (with all affected public partners) if a critically ill patient, accompanied by DOT Category A waste, needs to be transferred to another facility. The mere facts that the patient may be crossing state lines or may need to bypass other healthcare facilities in route to the final destination are highly charged legal and political issues that are very difficult to navigate in real time and should be predetermined by engaging and planning with all public partners in advance of a bioemergency.

Finally, though most importantly, each healthcare system must work hand in hand with their local health department, EMS agencies, and other local health partners to ensure that working relationships exist that promote the exchange of information, collaboration, and exercising their individual responses to the point where the individual elements of their collective response are indistinguishable to the victims of a bioemergency.

Finance

Preparing for and responding to bioemergencies often comes with a very steep price tag. Models of care for isolating and treating patients infected with special pathogens typically reverse the normal staffing ratios of one physician and multiple nurses providing care to multiple patients to a model where upward of five clinicians per shift are dedicated to a single patient. For healthcare systems that do not commonly activate their hospital incident command systems, the operation of a fully staffed command center (and contemporaneously backfilling command staff members' day-to-day roles where necessary) is exponentially more expensive than ordinary healthcare operations. Finally, when a bioemergency also requires the use of disposable personal protective equipment, costs will exceed most expectations. For example, responding to a patient under investigation while accounting for command center staff, equipment, supplies, and personal protective equipment can cost a healthcare system upward of $10,000 per shift during the diagnostic phase (without accounting for training in advance of such an activation) and $10,000–$20,000 or more per day of treatment for confirmed patients thereafter [3].

Considering the cost of preparing for and responding to a bioemergency at the onset of a healthcare system's bioemergency preparations, a healthcare system should establish a dedicated cost center to track expenses. This should be done in compliance with organizational, local, state, and federal requirements with an eye toward justifying expenditures and maximizing reimbursements.

Screening

While understanding that responding to bioemergencies is financially costly, the greatest cost to a healthcare system related to bioemergencies must always remain the safety of patients and staff. Therefore, when preparing for bioemergencies, healthcare systems should concentrate on two particular areas of concern: (i) managing points of entry and (ii) providing safe treatment. First, a healthcare system must determine all points of entry to their healthcare system (e.g., via an emergency department, satellite clinic, long-term care facility) and the likelihood of entry via one of those points of entry. Second, each healthcare system should identify the access points within each of those points of entry (e.g., how many ways can a patient or threat enter each of your facilities – ambulance bay, clinics, business office, loading docks, mail room, etc.). Within these points of entry, healthcare delivery systems must implement screening practices to rapidly identify and isolate persons with highly communicable diseases and promptly institute infection control precautions (e.g., providing patient with a face mask for those with respiratory illness). These screening practices can be syndromic based coupled with relevant epidemiological risk factors and universal travel screening or be more outbreak specific (e.g., screening for MERS) when an active outbreak is occurring anywhere in the world. By implementing screening during triage and before completing full patient evaluations in these settings can greatly reduce nosocomial transmission and assist in identifying and isolating potentially communicable disease persons. Additional screening questions should be guided by the background of the patient, the exposure history, and any relevant epidemiological factors.

To augment screening, visual aids such as posters and signs in appropriate languages depending on the patient population that is served should be strategically placed in clear line of sight for patients at the points of entry into the healthcare delivery system. These visual aids should contain infographics requesting patients for recent travel history and applicable signs/symptoms to apply infection control precautions (e.g., placing mask on the face if exhibiting respiratory symptoms) and to notify a healthcare provider.

Administrative and Operational Controls

Once a healthcare system has identified points of entry and developed screening protocols, the next step is to educate staff on implementation of those protocols and to test those protocols as often as possible. A simple best practice for testing the effectiveness of screening protocols is to conduct no-notice simulation exercise, also known as mystery patient drills where an actor(s) goes through the point of entry into the healthcare delivery system (e.g., emergency departments, clinics) unannounced [4]. Mystery patients should present with contagious symptoms and/or relevant travel histories and epidemiological risk factors, and the actor should take note of how quickly he/she is identified as a risk, provided personal protective equipment (PPE), and, ultimately, isolated.

Training clinicians on safely donning and doffing PPE and simulating the provision of care while donned are equally as important as training on screening protocols. Facilities must rely on their infection prevention and control departments as well as federal guidelines for PPE considerations – such as particular PPE ensembles and frequency of training. Compounding these challenges is that given the unique nature of each bioemergency, it is nearly impossible for regulatory bodies to proactively govern the realm of bioemergencies, making it difficult to ensure consistent compliance by covered entities.

Regulatory

Preparing for bioemergencies (in general) and operating biocontainment units (specifically) can leave healthcare regulatory personnel in very ambiguous and precarious situations. Most (if not all) of the regulations that guide our healthcare systems (and, therefore, our operation of biocontainment units) were not created with bioemergencies in mind. The 2014–2016 Ebola virus disease epidemic highlighted many ambiguities and areas of concern for which there are no explicit regulatory guidance and no case law. Consequently, facilities preparing for bioemergencies must perform a risk analysis of regulatory applicability to their units and give a great deal of thought to the legal implications of our decisions within these environments.

There are two examples which best illustrate our current state of ambiguity and the potential legal implications: (a) Department of Transportation (DOT) Pipeline and Hazardous Materials Safety Administration (PHMSA) regulations/guidelines applicable to the treatment of Ebola virus disease waste prior to closing the primary bag of waste and (b) decisions impacting standards of care for patients under investigation and patients with a confirmed highly communicable special pathogen.

During the 2014–2016 Ebola virus disease epidemic, healthcare facilities without access to on-site autoclaves were required to "treat" Ebola suspected waste prior to have the waste removed from their healthcare facilities. While the final stages of packaging and transport regulations were relatively explicit, the method pursuant to which a facility treated waste at the point of origin was unclear. DOT PHMSA "Guidance on the Proper Packaging of Ebola Suspected Waste" required the preparer "prior to closure, [to] treat potentially contaminated waste with an U.S. Environmental Protection Agency (EPA)-registered hospital disinfectant" [5]. Specifics on how to adequately treat said waste or the safest or preferred methodology were not provided. From an operational perspective, there were two options: spraying the waste with disinfectant or otherwise adding disinfectant sufficient to cover the waste. When making a determination as to whether or not spraying the entire contents of the primary bag resulted in a risk outweighing the benefit of said spraying, a facility had to conduct a facility-specific risk assessment that considered at least the following: (i) How much liquid spray is necessary to treat the contaminated waste? (ii) Will that amount of liquid significantly increase the weight of the primary bag? (iii) Will that additional weight (or will the liquid – in general) pose a greater risk to healthcare workers subsequently attempting to maneuver that waste? (iv) What is the risk of the liquid spray winding up on the floor of the hot zone and does that increase the likely of slipping and falling? Depending on the resources available and the particular environment in which your facility was operating, the results of your risk assessment and the subsequent manner in which you treated waste at the point of origin varied widely [6].

Another example of the ambiguous and uncomfortable environment in which bioemergencies operate relates to the proper standard of care for PUIs and patients with a confirmed special pathogen. The moral and ethical dilemmas that bioemergencies (in particular Ebola virus disease) pose have not been on the collective mind of the United States' healthcare system since the AIDS epidemic in the 1980s (i.e., the propriety of deviating from our ordinary standards of care for a certain population of patients – resulting in lower standards of care – based solely on the inherent risks to the healthcare workers providing treatment).

The common standard of care for confirmed patients with Ebola virus disease seems to be one of delaying invasive procedures until the patient is less contagious. Additionally, there are many procedures that would potentially generate body fluids in such copious amounts (or are otherwise deemed to pose such a high risk to healthcare workers) that the general sentiment is to withhold that level care despite the fact that identical care would be provided to the same patient but for his/her confirmed special pathogen.

These lesser standards of care pose obvious ethical and moral issues but could also pose significant legal issues. This medical malpractice component would be even further complicated if care is withheld from a PUI (rather than a patient with a confirmed special pathogen). If the PUI is subsequently ruled out for the special pathogen (which served as the basis for withholding the care) and the patient suffered harm as a result of being provided a lower standard of care, the question of the reasonability of withholding that care would seemingly always be a question of fact for a jury.

Accreditation

In seeming direct contrast to the limited known regulatory applicability of preparing for bioemergencies and operating biocontainment units, from an accreditation perspective, preparation for bioemergencies will be evaluated against the Joint Commission (Joint Commissions) Emergency Management Standards and the Centers for Medicare and Medicaid Services (CMS) final rule for emergency preparedness requirements for Medicare- and Medicaid-participating providers and suppliers [7]. Additionally, the operation of our biocontainment units (including satellite labs, on-unit autoclaves, etc.) will be evaluated against the same Joint Commission and CMS standards and conditions of participation that already govern the operation of our hospitals.

Conclusion

Preparing for and safely and effectively responding to bioemergencies via an emergency management-based approach requires consistent communication, coordination, and collaboration across all administrative levels of a healthcare system. The 2014–2016 Ebola outbreak enabled NYC Health + Hospitals, the nation's largest municipal healthcare delivery system, to successfully receive and treat NYC's single confirmed case of Ebola at its Bellevue Hospital Center. This success is attributed in large part to many factors including a strong public health system, dedicated and well-trained team of medical experts, equipment and resources needed to safely and effectively manage and treat such patients and, perhaps most importantly, the meticulous coordination and preparation that occurred before and during these events as part of the administrative process.

The components of a successful, systematic administrative program that can be leveraged in times of a bioemergency include a strong leadership team, public health partnerships, financial infrastructure, administrative controls, operational controls, emergency management structure, travel screening, and regulatory and accreditation issues. While this chapter provides a general outline of some of the core aspects of preparing for bioemergencies, there are additional elements of preparation and response that every healthcare system must consider, all of which will be unique to their individual environments (see Table 3.1 for additional considerations).

Ultimately, administrative considerations when preparing for bioemergencies are human affairs decisions that demand confidence, craft, and resilience of all stakeholders, namely, the leaders entrusted with their well-being within their respective organizations. Invariably, organizations succeed or fail from the strengths they maintain or weaknesses they accept; bioemergencies are one crucible in the all-hazards landscape that empower them do so.

Table 3.1 Components of a systematic administrative program

Emergency management	HICS structure	Implements incident command structure Provides a comprehensive, all-hazards approach Marries resources Provides situational awareness
	Leadership team	Clear roles, accountable, empowered, dedicated Responsible for incident response plan development, implementation, and maintenance Responsible for frequent and clear lines of communication with internal (i.e., staff, healthcare workers) and external (i.e., visitors, general public) for situational awareness Manages and procures resources needed Handles media inquiries Protects patient privacy Creates a culture of transparency and order to chaos
	Public health partnerships	Local and State Department of Health Mortuary services agency for decedent management Emergency management services (EMS) for patient transport Local and state emergency management agency Federal public health agencies

(continued)

Table 3.1 (continued)

Finance	Financial infrastructure	Cost center to capture all related expenses Define all related additional expenses that may occur Define daily patient charge structure
Screening	Travel screening	Implementing outbreak-specific travel screening with associated signs and symptoms at all points of entry into healthcare delivery system Implementing universal travel screening with appropriate signs and symptoms
	Administrative controls	Recruits trained and competent staff for patient care team Health monitoring Offers continued training and education Routine training and drills to maintain readiness Compliance with any regulations Validates processes and procedures related to bioemergency event Ensures scrupulous adherence to processes and procedures through competency and assessment
	Operational controls	Checklists, procedures, processes, protocols, and standard operating procedures related to all aspects of patient care, staff workflow, waste management, etc. Equipment, resources, and infrastructure are in place for bioemergency event
Regulatory and accreditation		The Joint Commission Centers for Medicare and Medicaid Services Local regulations

References

1. Alves LF, Cagliuso N Sr, Dunne W. Building the bridge between healthcare emergency management and daily operations. J Bus Contin Emer Plan. 2015–2016;9(2):137–48.
2. New York State Homeland Security and Emergency Services. Emergency management – exercises – HSEEP (Homeland Security Exercise Evaluation Program) [Internet]. Dhses.ny.gov. 2017 [cited 14 February 2017]. Available from: http://www.dhses.ny.gov/oem/exercise/hseep.cfm.
3. Fox M. Cost to treat Ebola: $1 million for two patients [Internet]. NBC News. 2017 [cited 14 February 2017]. Available from: http://www.nbcnews.com/storyline/ebola-virus-outbreak/cost-treat-ebola-1-million-two-patients-n250986.
4. Madad S, Masci J, Cagliuso N, Allen M. Preparedness for Zika virus disease – New York City; 2006. Available from: https://www.cdc.gov/mmwr/volumes/65/wr/mm6542a2.htm?s_cid=mm6542a2_e.
5. PHMSA Pipeline and Hazardous Materials Safety Administration. Procedural guidance on the proper packaging of Ebola suspected waste [Internet]. 2017 [cited 14 February 2017]. Available from: https://www.phmsa.dot.gov/transporting-infectious-substances/procedural-guidance-proper-packaging-ebola-suspected-waste.
6. PHMSA Pipeline and Hazardous Materials Safety Administration. Transporting infectious substances safely [Internet]. Phmsa.dot.gov. 2017 [cited 14 February 2017]. Available from: https://www.phmsa.dot.gov/transporting-infectious-substances/transporting-infectious-substances-safely.
7. Federal Register / Vol. 81, No. 180 / Friday, September 16, 2016 / Rules and Regulations. Department of Health and Human Services. [Internet] [cited 14 February 2017]. Available from: https://www.gpo.gov/fdsys/pkg/FR-2016-09-16/pdf/2016-21404.pdf.

Communications in Times of Crisis: A Narrative

4

Taylor Wilson

Crisis Communicator The very title of my role during the time the University of Nebraska Medical Center and its clinical partner, Nebraska Medicine, spent caring for three patients with the Ebola virus indicated that the worst had already taken place. Those patients we treated in the Nebraska Biocontainment Unit had infected those who treated them and, in turn, those health-care workers had gone onto infect others in the Omaha community. From my viewpoint, *that* would be a crisis. That would be a situation in which no amount of crisis communication could soothe the nerves of a panicked public.

So in explaining how we handled communicating the situation at hand in the fall of 2014, I viewed my role, along with the half-dozen or so skilled colleagues who supported me, as a team of precrisis communicators. It was our job to make sure what was happening on campus was communicated in such a way that the 12,000 or so people working at the med center, along with the more than one million people who lived in the area surrounding Omaha, didn't view what was happening here as a crisis. Our team of skilled health-care workers, who had been training for this moment for nearly 10 years and who were some of the most prepared people in the world to handle a disease like Ebola, had the situation well under control. Nothing to worry about, no need to picture a zombie apocalypse-like Ebola outbreak. These folks had their methods, they had their protocols, and you could trust them to keep themselves and the rest of the community safe.

Fortunately, because all of the above was true, my job was easy.

T. Wilson (✉)
Media Relations Sr. Coordinator, Nebraska Medicine, Omaha, NE, USA
e-mail: twilson@nebraskamed.com

A. Hewlett, A. R. K. Murthy (eds.), *Bioemergency Planning*,
https://doi.org/10.1007/978-3-319-77032-1_4

Preparation

The process of preparing for what was about to happen here when our first patient arrived actually started years before that date in early September of 2014. The daily and weekly communications within the organization laid a solid foundation that was beneficial when it came time to communicate the fact that Ebola virus was purposely being brought to our doorstep.

Those who came before me and many of those with whom I worked during our time caring for patients with Ebola were former journalists like I was. The past and present practice of the media relations team had been to share our medical experts with the media often. The infectious disease physicians who were regularly interviewed about everything from the flu to the bacteria on cell phones were familiar with the process and, in many cases, comfortable with it. However, few of them ever imagined that an interview with the local NBC affiliate about our room-disinfecting robot would ever prove useful when Ebola would thrust them into the national spotlight, but that is exactly what happened. Our experts who soon would be interviewed by NBC, CNN, and MSNBC, just to name a few, would be much more comfortable when a camera's record light came on because they had been there before. Of course the magnitude was different, but they had done interviews for years, and that certainly played a role in how comfortable they were while becoming a part of our precrisis communication plan.

In addition to preparing our experts, the years of media interviews they, and other UNMC and Nebraska Medicine colleagues, had engaged in also served another purpose. The repository of community goodwill that the med center had built up in the years prior to caring for patients with Ebola can't be underestimated. Obviously, these interviews weren't the sole reason the med center was so favorably viewed by the community – the medical miracles and research breakthroughs taking place here over decades certainly are the driving force here – but being a constant and reliable resource for media interviews which paint that positive picture of the great things happening here also played a major role. In other words, the community trusted us.

Of course, when it comes to something like Ebola, trust can erode quickly. We knew we had to communicate clearly, concisely, and transparently. So when representatives from the US Department of State visited the Nebraska Biocontainment Unit in August 2014 to determine its readiness to handle a situation like this, we viewed it as an opportunity. It was an opportunity to remind the media and the public that the unit existed, that the people who worked here had been training for years to treat a patient with a highly hazardous communicable disease like Ebola, and that there was a very real possibility that a patient with that very disease could be treated here in the very near future.

It was also an opportunity to stockpile the media resources we already had related to the NBU. Over the years photos and videos were taken of the NBU team conducting drill after drill. We had photos and video of the team members, of the personal protective equipment they would be wearing, and of the environment in which they would be working. So while we invited local media to come visit with our experts and get fresh video of the NBU immediately after the State Department visit, we knew there would likely be a demand from national media for the resources we had on file should we treat an actual patient with Ebola in the coming weeks. We placed those files online in a Dropbox folder and waited.

Ebola in Nebraska

It was just after Labor Day in 2014 when we received notice that the first Ebola patient to be treated in the NBU would arrive soon. The Serious Communicable Diseases Unit at Emory University in Atlanta was already treating the first two US patients with Ebola, so now it was our turn.

As was almost always the case during times of crisis, our communication team was pulled into the meeting involving the highest-level executives at the med center, along with Dr. Phil Smith, the medical director of the Nebraska Biocontainment Unit and the man who was the driving force behind the creation of the unit in 2005. We discussed first steps in announcing the arrival of the patient and laid out our plan to accommodate what we knew would be a large local and national media presence.

I will never forget what happened during that meeting. I had no idea what was about to be thrust upon me, what it would mean for my future career, and how it would shape my life in ways I couldn't possibly have expected. The funny thing is, to this day, I don't think I've asked anyone why or how what was about to happen actually transpired the way in which it did.

A brief bit of background info: Nebraska Medicine (the private, nonprofit healthcare system) and UNMC (the publicly funded medical school) work hand in hand but are two distinctly separate organizations. UNMC has a PR team, and Nebraska Medicine has a marketing team. We work jointly on many projects, but there were people in that room attending that meeting who essentially do the same thing I do, both for the hospital and for the medical school. However, it was this moment at this meeting that I believe proved to be crucial to the success of our communication plan in the weeks and months to come. Not because of who was chosen to lead the communication effort but because the dual nature of our communication teams can sometimes create confusion when the media is making contact with us.

Nebraska Medicine's VP of communication said we would have a singular point of contact for all things related to Ebola. It was at that point he turned to me and said "Taylor, you are going to be that person." I didn't see it coming and had no idea what it was to mean down the road. I did know it would be a huge responsibility, and the image of both organizations was at stake. After the initial shock wore off, it was time to carry out the plan.

Because we knew national media would soon be knocking on our door, we wanted to have a facility that could easily accommodate them along with their satellite trucks and also provide them with a nice view of the campus for their live reports. We have a crisis communication plan, which outlines the primary staging events for events like these. Unfortunately, both locations were unavailable because of construction. A third location also had another event going on, so we had to go with plan “D,” which was a building I wasn’t familiar with but turned out to be mostly optimal to fit the needs of the media. It had a large conference room with strong Internet connectivity, an area next to the building where satellite trucks could easily park without interfering with daily traffic and a large patio area which allowed news outlets to set up their cameras, erect tents over their cameras and reporters, and provide a clear view of the UNMC/Nebraska Medicine campus.

Now that we had identified our home base of media operations, we started to think about messaging and how we would make this announcement to the media and the public. We first conferred with our counterparts at Emory, since they had already been through this. We spoke with the CDC, the Douglas County Health Department, and Nebraska Department of Health and Human Services. We all needed to be on the same page with what we were saying about the patient – when he would arrive, how sick he was, etc. Of course, without a signed consent form, there was very little we could say about his condition because of HIPAA concerns. We would have to cross that bridge once the patient and his family members arrived here.

We invited local media to a press conference announcing we would soon be receiving our first patient. We briefed our experts on what kinds of questions to expect and shared the talking points we had developed in tandem with the other local entities previously mentioned. At the conclusion of that press conference is when the floodgates opened.

My phone rang, and rang, and rang. Texts came in by the dozens, as did emails. The names of major national news networks appeared in subject and signature lines. I recognized many of them. Fox News reporter John Roberts happened to be in Lincoln, NE, when this all happened and was on-site later that evening asking me questions. The deluge of requests was something I had never experienced before, but I instinctively started making a list on my iPad of requests, contact info, and deadlines. I made a point to personally respond to as many of these as humanly possible and did so as quickly as possible to let media know I was the point of contact. I began compiling a list of media members who wanted to be contacted with updates. That list was ultimately in the neighborhood of 330 outlets and individuals.

We had already decided to hold another press conference the following day since we would have more details about the patient and his transport to Omaha. I discovered media wanted a call-in number in order to listen to the press conference and ask questions if they couldn’t be there in person. We would later add streaming video to our press briefings to provide off-site media even better access to our message. We would also provide them with video and photos of the arrival of the patient and updates as often as possible.

We learned early on that it was important to provide these updates in accordance with something I call the “daily media appetite.” As a story like this breaks, the media appetite is nearly insatiable. Information comes out in a fire hose-like stream, and the media devours it. They want to learn everything they can about the situation. As the days and hours go on, the updates become less frequent, but no less important. We held more informal briefings in the days following the announcement of the arrival of our first patient. I would begin each day by reviewing the volume and type of requests I was receiving and respond accordingly. Who would be the best people to make available for interviews? When two nurses became ill while caring for an Ebola patient in Dallas, we had NBU nurses available to answer questions about the training, drills, and protocols that instilled a feeling of safety within the NBU.

We had a dozen or more press conferences during our time caring for and then subsequently monitoring patients for Ebola. At each one, we thought carefully about identifying the right spokespersons to tackle the topic at hand. We wanted someone caring for the patient, someone from hospital leadership and someone from university leadership. We often had an infectious disease expert along with either Dr. Smith or Dr. Angela Hewlett, the associate medical director of the Biocontainment Unit. At times other people were involved – the parents of our second patient were a part of one press conference. The leadership for the group for which our first patient worked joined us for a press conference after it was announced he would be transported to Nebraska for his care. The patient's wife held a press conference at one point, as did the patient himself when he was discharged from the NBU. We wanted to make sure we had the right people available to answer any question that might come up while, at the same time, not too many people to confuse the issue.

We also had to find creative ways to make our experts available. At the time, we didn't have an on-campus TV studio, so many of our experts did interviews via Skype or FaceTime. Some were over the phone, and some were via the satellite trucks where media camped out for days at a time. Some were off campus at local TV stations, which could relay the interviews to the national news networks. As you might imagine, caring for patients with Ebola is nearly a round-the-clock job by itself. Add to that the emotional burden of media interviews, and it quickly became clear we would need a "deep bench" to respond to the flurry of requests we were receiving.

Fortunately, we had a lot of experts willing to pitch in. I would triage the requests and pair our experts with media requests. Even our interim president at the time, Dr. Bradley Britigan, himself an infectious disease specialist, pitched in and did several interviews when needed. After being embedded with our Biocontainment Unit team for a period of time, I pinch hit and did interviews for outlets when I knew everyone was just too tired or too busy to do it themselves. In other words, media burnout is very real. You need to know your team's strengths, areas of expertise, and just how deep your bench is.

I can't underestimate how important a firm grasp of technology is throughout this process. Because this story got worldwide attention, I received requests for interviews or information at all hours of the day and night. I quickly learned I needed *all* of my information about this subject everywhere I was going to be, whether it was at my desk, at home, in my car or what quickly became my office away from the office, the NBU itself.

At the outset of all of this, I was working in the media center we had set up so I could quickly walk out the door and answer questions face-to-face. As time went on and most media outlets departed campus, I discovered the best place to be was working side by side with the people caring for the patients in the NBU. A "command center" was set up across the hall from the actual unit itself. This was where the caregivers held meetings, had lunch, and conducted conference calls with medical experts from around the world. This would soon become my office, where I would plug in my laptop and get face-to-face answers about questions the media had and would find subjects for live and taped interviews from major networks and local media as well. I can't emphasize how important it was to be physically close to the folks who were doing the heavy lifting medically. It's much easier to determine who is available and how prepared they are for an interview and to stay up to date on the condition of the patient. That physical closeness also translated in some cases to emotional closeness. The people with whom I was working learned to trust me and take my advice as time wore on.

Much of my advice came in the form of letting them know we need to address questions sooner rather than later. I always referred to this as a "culture of proactivity." We not only needed to respond in a timely manner but, in many cases, needed to have the responses prepared before the questions came. "No comment" is never an option as is putting your head in the sand and thinking the questions will go away. Doing that is the best way to quickly lose control of a situation and to have misinformation spread like wildfire, instead of the transparent truth, which you need to be sharing. Responding in a timely and transparent manner with answers that satisfy the daily media appetite not only allows you to have factual information shared in the media; it also establishes a strong relationship with media members because they recognize you as a trusted source they can rely on for frequent updates.

Having said all this, your experts need to know that it is ok to say "I don't know, but I will find that information for you." It's also ok to say "I can't share that information right now," as long as you have a valid reason for doing so. Patient confidentiality was often a reason for us being unable to share information, but we also had agreements in place with certain drug manufacturers that prohibited us from divulging information about which experimental treatments we were using.

Along with frequency and transparency, we also had contingency plans in place for our messages. In many cases, circumstances were changing rapidly due to patient condition and preparedness for transport. We had separate messaging prepared depending on when and if we received patient/family consent to share information about a patient's condition. We realized that once people within our organization learned about the possible arrival of a patient, that internal information could quickly become external. We worked closely with our internal communication team to share messaging nearly simultaneously so our internal colleagues and external audience (the media and public) received the same message at the same time.

In order to be so flexible with messaging, we had to be able to rapidly share it with our executive team and medical leadership as well. We developed texting and email groups to quickly gain approval of messaging, both internal and external. However, and I can't stress this enough, another aspect of our plan that helped it succeed was the fact that leadership trusted the communication team to do its job. I was allowed to craft daily patient updates by working closely with the patients' families and then talking to medical leadership about what they wanted to share at the time. I also handled most of the social media posts, responding to questions on Twitter and Facebook and even seeking out questions and misinformation on the social media sites of other media outlets. Having a frequent and accurate voice in the social media conversation was also extremely helpful in allowing our communication plan to succeed.

Being a former reporter myself, it was almost second nature to know what kind of information the media would be interested in. Anything that is *new* information, no matter how small, is big to the media. We had a photo of one of our patients wearing a Nebraska Cornhuskers' t-shirt that one of the doctors had given him. That was like gold to the media. The media also wants readily available content – the previously mentioned photos and videos we provided on Dropbox along with live video streams and video sound bites and b-roll are also heavily favored by newsrooms with ever-decreasing budgets that can't afford to send staff members to cover the story but still want to include it in their broadcasts. Anything that seems like insider information is also a big deal. Photos from inside the NBU taken of the staff members were very popular, along with exclusive interviews. The outlets with the reporters that knew the right questions to ask often ended up with interviews no one else had.

So what shouldn't you do? It seems simple, but I still see large organizations respond in times of crisis in one of several ways. It's often deadly to start crafting your message when the questions are already coming. You have to get ahead of the crisis, have the answers, have the people available to provide the answers, and anticipate the follow-up questions.

Some organizations still think the "no comment" comment absolves them of responsibility, and the crisis will just go away. As I mentioned earlier, this technique just allows the media, the public, or the bloggers to start making up their own narrative. That rarely ends well for the organization which relies on that technique.

Failing to respond in a timely fashion can also be deadly when media outlets are putting stories online and on social media often before a daily broadcast or publication. When a reporter is asking questions, you always need to ask what their deadline is, or the story may pop up online without input or perspective from your organization.

Conclusion

By the time the Ebola crisis had tapered off, the name of our organization had been mentioned online, on air, and in print nearly 60,000 times. We had a potential print and broadcast audience approaching one billion people. We fulfilled hundreds of interview requests and still receive them as we continue to lead the way in training other caregivers on the best methods to treat patients with highly hazardous communicable diseases. Communications truly requires a team-based approach, and being prepared to handle a wide variety of media encounters will be beneficial for an organization in a time of crisis.

Key Points for Communications in Times of Crisis

Always:

- Create a precrisis communication plan.
- Share information internally before media release.
- Identify a location for media staging.
- Stockpile media resources.
- Identify multiple experts and prepare them for interviews.
- Craft media messaging early.
- Assemble a comprehensive communication team, but create a single point of contact for media inquiries.
- Always be proactive, open, and transparent with the media.
- Provide timely updates to the media and internal partners.
- Keep in close contact with the direct patient care providers.
- Maintain the ability to be flexible with messaging as patient conditions change.
- Utilize and respond to social media.

Never:

- Wait until the patient arrives to craft your message.
- Use the term "no comment."
- Fail to respond to the media in a timely fashion.

5 Strategies for Waste Management and Decontamination

John J. Lowe and Katelyn Jelden

Introduction

Caring for patients with highly hazardous communicable diseases (HHCDs) presents unique challenges in clinical as well as nonclinical activities, including the safe management of waste contaminated with infectious pathogens. Medical waste generated during the care of a patient with a HHCD, along with the environment where the patient care cared for, pose an increased risk to healthcare, environmental service, and waste-handling workers due to characteristics of HHCDs which may include high morbidity and mortality, high communicability, and low infectious dose. Medical waste contaminated with or suspected of being contaminated with a HHCD pathogen should be collected, packaged, stored, and disposed of in a manner that adheres to regulatory guidance for packaging, storing, transporting, and disposing of waste. Environmental decontamination of the patient care area is also of utmost importance and should occur in a manner that utilizes optimal infection control protocols and procedures.

Prompted by the unprecedented 2014–2016 Ebola outbreak, US hospitals prepared for patients presenting with Ebola virus disease (EVD) and other HHCDs, known and unknown, informed by guidance and training provided by the Centers for Disease Control and Prevention (CDC) and hospitals that had successfully cared for patients with EVD (NETEC.org). Approaches for HHCD waste management vary within a national network of ~47 hospitals designated as Ebola treatment centers or federally designated as regional Ebola and other special pathogen treatment centers

J. J. Lowe (✉)
Department of Environmental and Occupational Health, College of Public Health, University of Nebraska Medical Center, Omaha, NE, USA
e-mail: jjlowe@unmc.edu

K. Jelden
College of Medicine, University of Nebraska Medical Center, Omaha, NE, USA

A. Hewlett, A. R. K. Murthy (eds.), *Bioemergency Planning*,
https://doi.org/10.1007/978-3-319-77032-1_5

[1]. In a survey of these centers, only 11 of 47 hospitals designated as Ebola treatment centers reported the capability to sterilize EVD-associated waste on-site using an autoclave or incinerator. The remaining Ebola treatment centers surveyed developed procedures to package medical waste and partnered with a certified waste vendor to transport this waste for incineration, at an enormous cost. In a follow-up survey completed by these centers in the spring of 2016, all 32 respondents reported having written protocols for routine hygiene (i.e., daily cleaning) of their HHCD isolation unit including surface cleaning and disinfection processes [2]. Nearly all (31/32) had written protocols for the final decontamination of the HHCD isolation unit and of medical devices, and all required training for personnel involved in decontamination. Regarding liquid waste disposal, 10 of 33 centers planned to solidify and dispose of liquid waste as solid waste, 4 centers planned to flush liquid waste down the toilet with no disinfectant, and 25 centers planned to treat the liquid waste with a disinfectant then flush the toilet. Incorporating lessons learned during several US hospitals' experience caring for patients with EVD, this chapter will discuss various methods hospitals can adopt to safely and effectively manage medical waste potentially contaminated with HHCD pathogens along with decontamination of patient care areas.

Medical Waste Regulation

Waste materials produced during the care of a patient with an HHCD known or reasonably suspected to contain infectious pathogens are subject to local, state, and federal procedures and regulations regarding medical waste packaging and disposal [3]. Infectious waste substances determined by the US Department of Transportation (DOT) to be "capable of posing an unreasonable risk to health, safety, and property when transported in commerce" are regulated as hazardous materials under US DOT Hazardous Materials Regulations (Hazardous Materials Regulations [HMR]; 49 CFR parts 171–180) when transported by air, highway, rail, or water [4]. Infectious medical waste is classified as Category A or Category B infectious substances [5]. Category A infectious substances are known or suspected to be contaminated with a pathogen that causes disease "in a form capable of causing permanent disability or life threatening or fatal disease in an otherwise healthy humans or animals when exposure occurs," while Category B waste is *not* in a form capable of causing permanent disability, life threatening, or fatal disease, i.e., regulated medical waste produced in routine care. Infectious materials produced in the care of patients with HHCDs, e.g., Ebola, are considered Category A waste and require HMR compliance unless a special permit has been granted.

Infectious substances produced during patient care include, but are not limited to, medical equipment, sharps, linens, and used healthcare products (such as soiled absorbent pads or dressings, kidney-shaped emesis pans, portable toilets, used personal protective equipment (gowns, masks, gloves, goggles, face shields, respirators, booties, etc.), or by-products of cleaning) contaminated or suspected of being contaminated [7]. Materials excepted of Category A regulations include (1) human remains transported for cremation, burial, or medical research at a college, hospital, or laboratory; (2) linens or medical equipment in compliance with the Occupational Safety and Health Administration (OSHA) blood-borne pathogens standard that is intended for reuse, cleaning, or refurbishment (not including medical equipment which is to be disposed of); (3) waste produced during emergency medical service transport and care of a patient suspected or known to be infected with an HHCD (HMR apply upon arrival to a site where the emergency vehicle will be decontaminated); and (4) material that has been treated to inactivate or entirely remove the pathogen (e.g., autoclave or incineration) [7]. Overall, Category A infectious substances require stringent packaging and treatment to completely inactivate pathogens or incineration to be transported for disposal. The HMR and resources from the US DOT and CDC offer additional information pertaining to infectious medical waste regulation [3, 5, 7, 8].

Clinically Relevant Pathogens Regulated as Category A Infectious Substances [6]

- Crimean-Congo hemorrhagic fever virus
- Ebola virus
- Guanarito virus
- Hantaan virus
- Hendra virus
- Junin virus
- Kyasanur Forest disease virus
- Lassa virus
- Machupo virus
- Marburg virus
- Monkeypox virus
- Nipah virus
- Omsk hemorrhagic fever virus

Medical Waste Suspected of HHCD Contamination

During the initial assessment of a patient suspected to have an HHCD (i.e., person under investigation [PUI]), whether medical waste is subject to HMR is contingent on patient diagnosis. Medical waste suspected to be contaminated with a HHCD pathogen may be preemptively packaged and handled as a Category A infectious substance before a diagnosis is determined. However, waste cannot be reclassified as Category B waste once Category A packaging procedures have commenced and significant expenses have been associated with the transport of Category A infectious substances. Until test results confirm or refute the HHCD diagnosis, medical waste generated in care may be sequestered for later packaging and transport. It is suggested to dedicate a secure, separate room for waste storage where materials can be placed within large, contained (i.e., covered) wheeled carts for ease of transport. Carts should be lined with absorbent material layered proximally to disposable plastic (or water-resistant material) and labeled with a note indicating that terminal cleaning will be necessary following use. Medical waste generated in the care of a PUI should be contained within two plastic bag layers, placed inside the carts, and held within the room until a confirmatory diagnosis is received. If a HHCD diagnosis is ruled-out, the medical waste may be handled in accordance with local waste management ordinances. If a HHCD diagnosis is confirmed, Category A waste management procedures (e.g., on-site sterilization or off-site transport for incineration) should ensue. Medical waste generated in an ambulance during emergency medical service transport of a patient suspected or confirmed to have an HHCD may be left at the receiving hospital, who should assume responsibility for managing the waste according to the HMR if determined to be a Category A infectious substance [7].

On-Site Waste Sterilization

Category A infectious waste that has been treated to inactivate or remove the pathogen is excepted in the HMR and *not* considered to be regulated medical waste or hazardous material under federal law, yet HHCD-associated waste is regulated by local, state, and OSHA requirements [3]. As a hospital prepares to care for a patient with a HHCD, it should be predetermined whether infectious materials generated during care will be sterilized on-site at the medical facility or transported as Category A infectious substance for off-site disposal. Hospitals that cared for patients with EVD have implemented on-site waste sterilization techniques using an appropriate, validated autoclave [9, 10]. Additionally, waste may be incinerated on-site and the remaining contents, i.e., ash, disposed of following hospital protocols and state and local regulations [3]. Purchase and installation of an autoclave or incineration system costs approximately US $100,000 [1]. Other methods of pathogen inactivation, such as chemical sterilization, have not been standardized with medical waste, would require worker safety assessment, and may involve other federal safety regulations [3]. Sterilization procedures should be developed to accommodate all textures found within a HHCD patient care unit (e.g., linens, mattresses, pillows), noting unnecessary materials, such as privacy curtains, should be removed prior to patient occupation to reduce cleaning and autoclave burdens [9].

The packaging of infectious waste for autoclave sterilization should be initiated in a contained and contaminated zone, i.e., the patient care room or doffing zone where the waste is generated. In units that cared for patients with EVD, primary packaging of waste was completed by patient care staff wearing PPE identical to the level worn during patient care (including at minimum a fluid-resistant gown or suit, a N95 respirator or powered air-purifying respirator, nitrile gloves, a face shield, and booties) as demonstrated in Fig. 5.1 [9]. It was reasoned that waste management performed by patient care staff (e.g., nurses, medical care technicians) would reduce

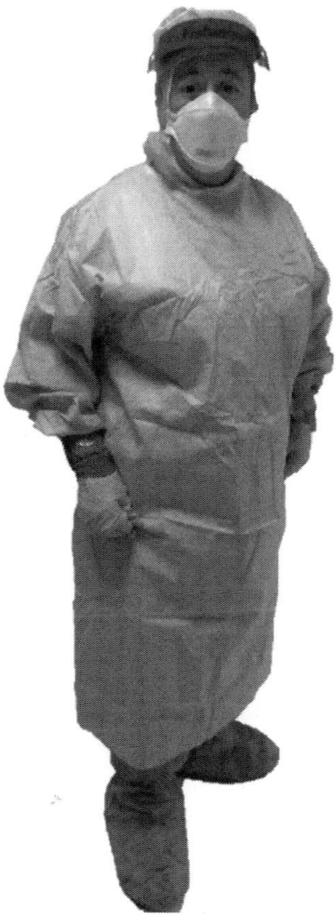

Fig. 5.1 Example of personal protective equipment (PPE) level worn by waste handlers to autoclave or package medical waste as Category A infectious substance for disposal. The full precaution PPE level is identical to patient care standards

the overall number of individuals in contact with contaminated materials while utilizing staff already experienced in high-level PPE donning and doffing. Contaminated sharps should be placed inside an appropriate disposable sharps container for autoclave sterilization. Solid waste should be collected in leakproof, clear autoclave bags and loosely gooseneck closed with autoclave tape when reaching ~75% capacity [9]. It is recommended autoclave bags be placed inside waste bins with a slightly smaller volume than the autoclave bags, so that when a waste bin appears filled, the autoclave bag within is holding ~75% capacity or less and bags cannot be overfilled. The outside surface of each autoclave bag should be wiped with an EPA-registered hospital disinfectant prior to removal from the patient room or doffing area. As large volumes of waste are generated during the care of patients with HHCDs and autoclave capacity is limited, it is recommended that surplus, unsterilized waste bags are stored in a separate room, preferably in close proximity to the patient care area, within plastic/absorbent-lined wheeled carts until autoclaved. Staff responsible for autoclaving the biohazardous solid waste can roll the carts containing waste to the autoclave for sterilization rather than carry exposed waste bags. Preferably, an autoclave should be located near the patient care area to reduce potential contamination and exposure during transport.

Autoclave setting parameters and procedures used for waste sterilization should be validated with local and state health authorities as well as partnering with waste-handling and transportation vendor. Validation procedures might incorporate biological and chemical indicators placed within realistic waste loads (~75% autoclave bag capacity) containing various texture types found in the HHCD care setting such as PPE, bed linens, scrubs, paper, and plastic (e.g., suction canisters, sharps containers) under both dry and water-saturated conditions [11]. Of note, one study found that manufacturer-recommended settings were likely insufficient to inactivate pathogens at the center of waste loads simulating those found in the patient care environment [11], and autoclave parameters such as temperature or treatment length may need to be adjusted to meet the sterilization demands of HHCD medical waste. When actively caring for a patient with a HHCD, autoclave function should be evaluated via validation procedures (at minimum biological and chemical indicators) as least once per 24-h period. When the HHCD isolation unit is unoccupied, autoclave validation should occur at least once per week and in accordance with manufacturer guidelines. Autoclave validation results should be stringently documented, both during activation and inactivation periods.

A pass-through autoclave is preferable for the sterilization of medical waste, as bags can be loaded into the autoclave on a designated "dirty" or contaminated side by staff in full PPE. After the sterilization cycle is complete, the sterilized waste bags are unloaded from a separate door on the opposite "clean" or non-contaminated side of the autoclave. The pass-through autoclave "Bioseal" feature prevents biological cross-contamination across dirty and clean sides. Portable autoclaves may also be valuable for medical waste sterilization although they may be limited by rate and capacity processing of large waste volumes [9]. All staff that operate an autoclave should be trained in autoclave protocols as well as donning and doffing PPE to demonstrable competencies [12].

Medical facilities should develop procedures to sterilize and/or dispose of diverse contaminated materials from the patient care area. Certain items cannot withstand or should not be subjected to the temperatures and pressures of an autoclave, such as radioactive materials; combustible, flammable, volatile, or highly corrosive liquids; liquids sealed in a container; materials contaminated with chemotherapeutic agents; and some plastics [13, 14]. At least one facility that cared for patients with EVD autoclaved healthcare worker scrubs for reuse [9]. Following autoclave sterilization, scrubs were placed inside a hospital soiled linen receptacle for additional washing. Autoclave-sterilized waste is not considered to be regulated medical waste or a hazardous material under federal law but remains subject to local, state, and OSHA regulation. For instance, a hospital experienced in caring for patients with EVD placed sterilized EVD-associated waste from the clean side of the autoclave into a biohazard bag that lined a primary watertight receptacle and rigid outer packaging for transport as Category B regulated medical waste [9]. Although not requiring a DOT special permit, this EVD-associated waste was tracked to the incineration facility similarly to Category A infectious substances.

Hospitals planning to use an autoclave for medical waste sterilization during the care of a patient with a HHCD should develop alternate strategies for managing waste if their autoclave(s) becomes inoperative. Hospitals federally designated as regional Ebola and other special pathogen treatment centers have invested in two independently functioning autoclaves to increase waste processing capacity and rate while serving as backup if one autoclave was to become nonfunctional [11]. It is recommended that autoclave electrical and mechanical components are accessible on the non-contaminated side for repairs. Other autoclaves may be available for emergency use at a medical campus if waste can be safely and securely transported to the autoclave site or an autoclave transported into the HHCD isolation unit. Furthermore, plans should be developed to package and transport medical waste as Category A infectious substances for disposal at an off-site waste management facility, details of which will be discussed in the following section.

Packaging Category A Waste for Transportation and Off-Site Disposal

Category A infectious substances are subject to the US DOT's HMR [4]when transported by air, highway, rail, or water [8]. Strict adherence to the HMR is required, but if discrepancies from the HMR are necessitated, a special permit may be requested under 49 CFR § 107.105 that may be granted by the DOT if an applicant can demonstrate alternative packaging that will meet or surpass the level of safety required by the HMR or consistent with public interest if no required safety level exists [15]. This text should not be used to determine HMR compliance, and further details of Category A infectious substance packaging can be found in the HMR and through DOT and CDC resources [7, 8, 15–17]. Staff who package medical waste should wear full PPE, similar or identical to the level of PPE worn during patient care activities, and be adequately trained and demonstrate competency to don and doff the PPE [12].

Medical waste placed inside primary biohazard bags and sharps containers should not be compressed or filled beyond two-thirds full to reduce risk of pathogen aerosolization and ensure bags will fit into subsequent 55-gallon packaging containers. It is critically important to not overfill waste bags, as overfilling would require staff to redistribute contaminated materials, which presents an unnecessary exposure risk to waste handlers.

To begin packaging medical waste as Category A infectious substances, solid materials (e.g., materials from patient care, PPE) should be placed inside a watertight plastic bag (i.e., biohazard bag) that may weight no more than 10 kg (22 lbs.) when filled [15]. This primary plastic bag must be 175 L (46 gal) or smaller, have an impact resistance of 165 g and a tearing resistance of 480 g in both the parallel and perpendicular planes, and be compatible with an EPA-registered hospital disinfectant. An EPA-registered hospital disinfectant must be added inside the primary plastic bag to treat potentially contaminated waste before the bag is removed from the patient's room or the doffing area, as required by the DOT Special Permit 16,279. Sharps placed inside an authorized sharps container should be sealed following instructions specific to that sharps container. Objects with sharp edges should be wrapped to prevent tearing/puncture of the plastic bag. The primary bag should be knotted or sealed to prevent liquid leakage, and the outside of the bag should be wiped with an EPA-registered hospital disinfectant. Next, the primary plastic bag should be placed inside a second watertight plastic bag with the primary bag's knot facing upward. The second plastic bag should be knotted or sealed ensuring the primary bag within does not obstruct closing. The outside of the second plastic bag (containing the first bag) should be wiped with an EPA-registered hospital disinfectant. Finally, the double-lined plastic waste bag should be placed inside a third layer of outer packaging, either a rigid United Nations standard or DOT-approved non-bulk packaging (i.e., 55 gallon cardboard container). If the outer packaging is composed of fiberboard, it should be triple walled with a 6 mm polyethylene plastic liner. Absorbent material sufficient to absorb any free liquid within the bags should be placed at the bottom of the outer package. Once the double-lined plastic waste bag is placed inside the outer packaging, the liner (if applicable) should be closed and the outer packaging also closed according to manufacturer instructions. The outside of the outer packaging should be wiped with an EPA-registered hospital disinfectant. In summary, infectious waste should be layered within (1) primary watertight plastic bag, (2) secondary watertight plastic bag, and (3) approved Category A rigid outer container.

The outer packaging must remain closed unless loading medical waste bags inside as multiple plastic bags may fit inside the outer packaging [15]. The medical facility must ensure the outer packaging is not leaking and has been appropriately sealed before the container is loaded into a transport vehicle for off-site disposal. The outer package must be marked with the United Nations number 2814 infectious substances, affecting humans. A shipping paper must accompany the shipment that includes key hazard information such as the United Nations number and proper shipping name, hazard class (i.e., Division 6.2 infectious), and emergency contact information. The partnering waste vendor must obtain a DOT Category A infectious substance special permit for transportation to an appropriate incineration facility [7]. The transport waste vendor must have an en route transport security plan and an emergency response plan in case of spills or other emergency situations [7].

Notably, medical facilities without autoclave or incinerator capabilities should be prepared to expend possibly millions of US dollars to ship Category A waste for disposal [1], as has been anecdotally noted by a hospital that cared for a patient with EVD. At the time of this writing, a very limited number of hazardous waste incinerator facilities in the US will accept Category A infectious substances associated with EVD, which will result in significant transport costs to dispose of Category A infectious substances that far exceed the cost of transport and disposal of regulated medical waste produced in routine patient care.

Liquid Waste

Copious amounts of liquid waste such as vomit, urine, blood, and feces may be generated during the care of a patient with a HHCD, as was seen while caring for patients with EVD that produced 9–10 L of liquid waste per day [9, 10]. Liquid waste disposal procedures must incorporate state and local regulations. Sanitary sewage systems are equipped to safely process liquid waste contaminated with special pathogens, and CDC guidance on managing liquid waste from patients with EVD does not recommend treating liquid waste with disinfectant [17]. No published data exists on the effectiveness of disinfectants against viruses in human waste, and no EPA-registered hospital disinfectant has been approved for use against viruses in feces, urine, or vomit in the toilet before disposal. It is also known that viruses will associate with particles and organic matter in patient waste to decrease the effectiveness of disinfectants [18]. However, hospitals that have cared for patients with EVD have treated liquid waste with an EPA-registered hospital disinfectant prior to flushing to alleviate concerns raised by staff from facility maintenance and plumbing as well as individuals from local public works [9, 10]. In the experience of one hospital, all EVD-contaminated liquid waste was placed in the toilet and an appropriate concentration of an EPA-registered hospital disinfectant (compatible with plumbing) added [9]. The liquid waste/disinfectant was held in the toilet for at least twice the manufacturer-recommended contact time (~10 min) before a rigid, nonporous closure was placed over the toilet for flushing. The toilet handles, seat, and lid surfaces were wiped with disinfectant. Liquid wastes from difficult to open containers, such as suction canisters, were not placed inside the toilet but were rather autoclaved on a liquid cycle setting. Medical facilities preparing to care for patients with HHCDs without an accessible, private toilet might consider the use of a covered bedside commode to collect liquid waste [18]. Some medical facilities add solidifier to commode contents to reduce risk of spills and dispose of the contents according to solid waste procedures. Bowel management systems may be useful to manage patients who are unstable, produce liquid stool, or are incapable of safely ambulating to the commode.

Laboratory Waste

Medical waste associated with a HHCD patient that is produced during laboratory procedures is subject to state and local regulation concerning disposal. Hospitals experienced in EVD care have set up point-of-care laboratories within isolated patient care units, so waste generated in the laboratory can be integrated into waste streams and appropriately autoclaved or packaged for off-site disposal. The laboratory waste generated from a PUI or patient with a HHCD is *not* subject to select agent regulations unless viable pathogen has been intentionally isolated from the waste [19]. Lastly, hospitals and laboratories that have cared for HHCD patients may not retain specimens from these patients, as "once patient care for the select agent infection has concluded, specimens become subject to the select agent regulations unless they are destroyed within seven calendar days of the conclusion of patient care" [19, 20].

Decontamination

Decontamination procedures should be developed for patient entry routes through the healthcare facility [21]. As a patient with an HHCD is transported from an entrance point to the isolation unit and until decontamination procedures are completed, access to the area should be entirely restricted to isolation unit staff wearing PPE at a level compatible with patient care. Immediately following patient admittance into the isolation unit, the floors, doors, and walls along the patient transport route should be immediately wiped and disinfected by isolation unit staff in full PPE. Solid waste and PPE produced while cleaning the patient entry route in the healthcare facility should join the solid waste stream generated from within the isolation unit.

Patients who present to the hospital for HHCD care may bring personal items that require pathogen inactivation before return or disposal, if necessary. In the experiences of hospitals caring for patients with EVD, several individuals were medically evacuated by air ambulance from West Africa carrying luggage in the form of clothing, currency, passports, electronics, etc. Items such as clothing and passports could be safely sterilized in the autoclave and were returned to patients or their family. Electronic items, such as cell phones, cameras, and laptops, could not be processed in the autoclave for risk of explosion and subsequent autoclave damage, so these items were soaked in an EPA-registered disinfectant and exposed to pathogen-inactivating doses of ultraviolet light before return to patients. Alternative sterilization methods for personal items might include treatment with gaseous chlorine dioxide or vaporized hydrogen peroxide.

Routine environmental cleaning and disinfection of the HHCD isolation unit surfaces and floors should be completed at least daily, preferably by healthcare workers in downtime when not completing patient care tasks. Thus, the number of individuals potentially exposed to the HHCD is limited, and access to the isolation unit is restricted to staff skilled in isolation unit procedures and PPE use (Fig. 5.2). Spill and bodily fluid cleanup procedures should minimize staff contact with infectious fluids. For instance, several layers of absorbent cloths may be gently laid on liquid spills and disposed of as solid waste. In this method, absorbent cloths may be laid on top of the fluid until the top layer appears dry, and then while only touching the top layer, the absorbent cloths can be scooped and disposed of as solid waste. Depending on the volume of the liquid spill, additional absorbent cloths may need to be laid on residual fluid and the procedure repeated. Using this approach, gloved staff hands should not directly contact the liquid spill but may do so instead with a dry cloth barrier. Healthcare worker scrubs and towels can be autoclaved and then washed through hospital laundry processes [9].

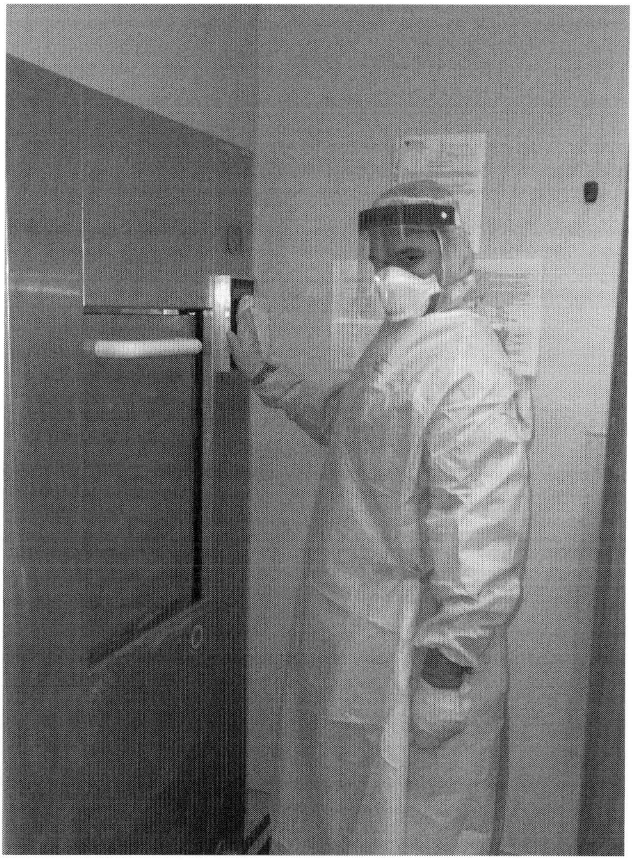

Fig. 5.2 Autoclave operator performing surface cleaning of the autoclave

HHCD isolation units should be terminally decontaminated following patient dismissal [22]. PPE worn by personnel completing terminal cleaning should match the level of PPE from patient care activities. Immediately following patient dismissal, linens and solid waste should be removed from the patient room and appropriately disposed. A hospital experienced in caring for patients with EVD reported restricting all personnel access to their isolation unit for 48 h while running high airflows of 15–19 high-efficiency particulate absorption-filtered air exchanges per hour to allow for viral desiccation. Staff who complete terminal cleaning should be trained specifically in handling materials contaminated with HHCDs (including PPE donning and doffing), and infection control personnel should observe terminal cleaning for quality control. The isolation unit floors should be mopped with a hospital grade disinfectant starting at the area least likely to be contaminated (e.g., the isolation unit entrance) and finishing in areas most likely to be contaminated (e.g., the patient room). All surfaces should be manually wiped with disinfectant under observation by infection control personnel (Fig. 5.3). Medical devices used during

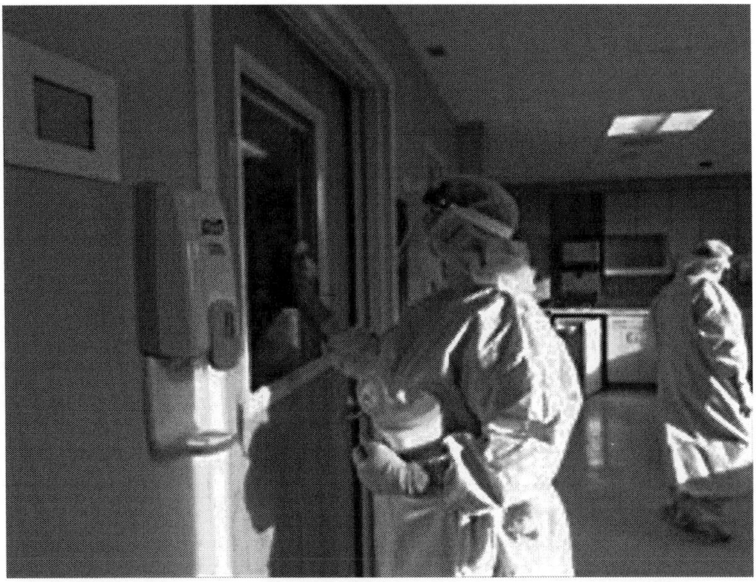

Fig. 5.3 Team-based approach to terminal decontamination of the patient care unit

patient care should be cleaned and terminally decontaminated following manufacturer recommendations. Non-touch disinfection processes, such as exposure with hydrogen peroxide vapor or UV light, may be included in final decontamination of the isolation unit and medical equipment after all surfaces have been manually disinfected. A second 48-h period of restricted access under high airflow may then be implemented for further pathogen desiccation, as was completed by a hospital experienced in EVD care. Following a second 48-h no-entry period, the isolation unit was deemed safe to enter without PPE. Following the decontamination protocol, environmental services staff may perform aesthetic cleaning to remove chemical residues on surfaces while wearing standard hospital cleaning PPE.

Lessons Learned and Recommendations

Experiences garnered by hospitals while caring for patients with EVD have provided key insights into the effective management of HHCD medical waste and appropriate decontamination strategies for patient care units. Of the many lessons learned, it is emphasized that high volumes of waste will be generated in the care of patients with HHCDs. Patients may be critically ill and will require large quantities of disposable medical materials. Moreover, generally two or more patient care staff wearing full PPE are omnipresent in the HHCD setting with limited abilities to wear this PPE for long durations (usually less than 4 h). PPE will likely compose the bulk of disposed medical waste. Additionally, building strong partnerships with local health authorities and biomedical waste vendors is invaluable to navigating HHCD waste management. Local, state, and federal rules, regulations, and guidelines pertaining to HHCD medical waste must be thoroughly understood and strictly followed. Finally, it is of utmost importance to document the occurrence of all procedures and protocols in HHCD medical waste management, such as autoclave validation results and Category A infectious substance manifest tracking to incineration facilities. The disposal of medical waste contaminated with HHCD pathogens and decontamination of patient care areas can be managed safely and effectively with adequate preparation by hospitals and collaborative work with partners in waste management and infection control.

References

1. Herstein JJ, Biddinger PD, Kraft CS, Saiman L, et al. Current capabilities and capacity of Ebola Treatment Centers in the United States. Infect Control Hosp Epidemiol. 2016;37(03):313–8.
2. Herstein JJ, Biddinger PD, Gibbs SG, Le AB, et al. High-level isolation unit infection control procedures. Health Security. 2017;15(5):519–26. https://doi.org/10.1089/hs.2017.0026
3. Centers for Disease Control and Prevention (CDC). Ebola-associated waste management. 2015. Retrieved January 16, 2017, from https://www.cdc.gov/vhf/ebola/healthcare-us/cleaning/waste-management.html.
4. United States Government. Hazardous Materials Regulations. 49 C.F.R. Parts 171–180. Available from: http://www.ecfr.gov/cgi-bin/text-idx?SID=eec3801875105d88488ca31976310098&mc=true&tpl=/ecfrbrowse/Title49/49CIsubchapC.tpl. Data current as of October 30, 2017. Accessed 16 January 16, 2017.
5. United States Department of Transportation (DOT). Transporting infectious substances safely. 2006. Retrieved January 16, 2017, from http://www.phmsa.dot.gov/pv_obj_cache/pv_obj_id_54AC1BCBF0DFBE298024C4C700569893C2582700/filename/Transporting_Infectious_Substances_brochure.pdf.
6. WHO. Guidance on regulations for the Transport of Infectious Substances 2007–2008. Available from: http://www.who.int/csr/resources/publications/biosafety/WHO_CDS_EPR_2007_2cc.pdf.
7. United States Department of Transportation (DOT), Pipeline and Hazardous Materials Safety Administration. Safety advisory: Packaging and handling Ebola virus contaminated infectious waste for transportation to disposal sites. 2014. Docket no. PHMSA–2014–0134, notice no. 14–04. Federal Registrar, 79(210), 64646. Available from: https://www.gpo.gov/fdsys/pkg/FR-2014-10-30/pdf/2014-25778.pdf. Accessed January 17, 2017.
8. United States Government. Definitions classification, packing group assignments and exceptions for hazardous materials other than class 1 and class 7. 49 C.F.R. Sect. 173.134. Available from: http://www.ecfr.gov/cgi-bin/text-idx?SID1/4e35d034b2154456059cd69b2893745df&node1/4se49.2.173_1134&rgn1/4div8. Accessed January 16, 2017.
9. Lowe JJ, Gibbs SG, Schwedhelm SS, Nguyen J, Smith PW. Nebraska biocontainment unit perspective on disposal of Ebola medical waste. Am J Infect Control. 2014;42(12):1256–7. https://doi.org/10.1016/j.ajic.2014.10.006.
10. Stephens DS, Ribner BS, Gartland BD, Feistritzer NR, Farley MM, Larsen CP, Fox JT. Ebola virus disease: experience and decision making for the first patients outside of Africa. PLoS Med. 2015;12(7):e1001857.
11. Garibaldi BT, Reimers M, Ernst N, Bova G, et al. Validation of autoclave protocols for the successful decontamination of Category A medical waste generated from the care of patients with serious communicable diseases. J Clin Microbiol. 2016;55:545–51. JCM-02161
12. Occupational Safety and Health Administration (OSHA), National Institute for Occupational Safety and Health (NIOSH), Environmental Protection Agency (EPA). Safe handling, treat-

ment, transport and disposal of Ebola-contaminated waste. 2016. Retrieved January 16, 2017, from https://www.osha.gov/Publications/OSHA_FS-3766.pdf.

13. CSULA Environmental Health and Safety Biosafety Office. Fact sheet: Using autoclaves safely. Retrieved January 16, 2017, from http://www.calstatela.edu/sites/default/files/groups/Environmental%20Health%20and%20Safety/autoclavefactsheet.pdf.
14. University of Ottawa Environmental Health and Safety Service. A guideline for the safe use of autoclaves. 2003. Retrieved January 16, 2017, from https://uwaterloo.ca/safety-office/sites/ca.safety-office/files/uploads/files/guideline-for-safe-use-of-autoclaves.pdf.
15. United States Department of Transportation (DOT). Procedural guidance on the proper packaging of Ebola suspected waste, DOT guidance for preparing packages of Ebola contaminated waste for transportation and disposal. Retrieved January 16, 2017, from http://phmsa.dot.gov/staticfiles/PHMSA/DownloadableFiles/Files/suspected_ebola_patient_packaging_guidance_final.pdf.
16. Centers for Disease Control and Prevention (CDC). Interim guidance for environmental infection control in hospitals for Ebola virus. 2015. Retrieved January 16, 2017, from https://www.cdc.gov/vhf/ebola/healthcare-us/cleaning/hospitals.html#seven.
17. Centers for Disease Control and Prevention (CDC). Procedures for safe handling and management of Ebola-associated waste. 2015. Retrieved January 16, 2017, from https://www.cdc.gov/vhf/ebola/healthcare-us/cleaning/handling-waste.html.
18. National Ebola Training and Education Center (NETEC). Waste management. Retrieved January 16, 2017, from http://netec.org/wp-content/uploads/2015/09/10-NETEC-Waste-Management.pdf.
19. National Ebola Training and Education Center (NETEC). Laboratory testing and safety. Retrieved January 16, 2017, from http://netec.org/wp-content/uploads/2015/09/14-NETEC-Laboratory.pdf.
20. Centers for Disease Control and Prevention (CDC). Interim Guidance Regarding Compliance with Select Agent Regulations for Laboratories Handling Patient Specimens Under Investigation or Confirmed for Ebola Virus Disease (EVD). 2015. Retrieved January 18, 2017, from https://www.cdc.gov/vhf/ebola/healthcare-us/laboratories/select-agent-regulations.html.
21. Lowe JJ, Olinger PL, Gibbs SG, Rengarajan K, et al. Environmental infection control considerations for Ebola. Am J Infect Control. 2015;43(7):747–9. https://doi.org/10.1016/j.ajic.2015.03.006.
22. Jelden KC, Gibbs SG, Smith PW, Schwedhelm MM, et al. Nebraska biocontainment unit patient discharge and environmental decontamination after Ebola care. Am J Infect Control, DOI. 2015;43(3):203–5. https://doi.org/10.1016/j.ajic.2014.12.005

Laboratory Processing of Specimens

6

Peter C. Iwen, Roxanne Alter, Vicki L. Herrera,
Anthony R. Sambol, Karen L. Stiles, and Steven H. Hinrichs

Introduction and Background

The laboratory processing of clinical specimens is an essential function for any hospital providing care for patients. Accordingly, laboratory administrators are required to have an operational laboratory that can provide not only accurate and reliable results but also an environment that is safe for the laboratory worker. Although low risk, any specimen has the potential to contain a pathogen that could cause a laboratory-acquired infection; thus whether supporting a small critical access hospital or a large acute care facility, the laboratory needs to be prepared to handle specimens with a potential to contain or known to contain a high-risk pathogen. These emerging high-risk pathogens (also defined as high-consequence pathogen [HCP] or risk group 4 [RG-4] pathogen) have the ability to cause serious or lethal human disease for which preventative or therapeutic interventions are not readily available.

The Ebola virus (EV) epidemic of 2014–2016 highlighted the need for medical facilities to enhance their capabilities to handle specimens that might contain a RG-4 pathogen [1]. In a recent survey of infectious diseases physicians, a question was asked as to where they think specimens with the potential to contain a RG-4 pathogen were tested. The results showed that <50% of these physicians surveyed had a clear understanding where this testing was performed. They suggested that laboratory testing was most likely performed off-site (38%) without describing where this might be or they were unsure where this testing was done (22%) [2]. In

P. C. Iwen (✉) · R. Alter · V. L. Herrera · A. R. Sambol · K. L. Stiles
Nebraska Public Health Laboratory, Department of Pathology and Microbiology,
University of Nebraska Medical Center, Omaha, NE, USA
e-mail: piwen@unmc.edu

S. H. Hinrichs
College of Medicine, Department of Pathology and Microbiology,
University of Nebraska Medical Center, Omaha, NE, USA

A. Hewlett, A. R. K. Murthy (eds.), *Bioemergency Planning*,
https://doi.org/10.1007/978-3-319-77032-1_6

a follow-up to this survey, a compilation of comments from these physicians showed that the clinical laboratory generated the second highest level of comments after personal protective equipment (PPE), suggesting that many unknowns still existed on how the laboratory supported the care of patients infected with a HCP [3]. Another study also showed significant discrepancies in guidance documents for clinical laboratories from both professional and government sources which exacerbate the difficulty and confusion inherent in dealing with an emerging infectious disease [4].

Since the EV epidemic, the Centers for Disease Control and Prevention (CDC) in collaboration with individuals from medical facilities in the USA and those from resource-limited areas in Africa where patients with Ebola virus disease (EVD) were treated developed guidance materials for medical facilities for the management of patients with EVD. These documents included information for the laboratory such as generalized protocols for PPE usage [5], the safe handling and management of infectious waste [6], the managing and testing of clinical specimens [7], and the collection, transport, and submission of specimens [8]. Although these documents were developed with EV in mind, they were compiled as generalized to be useful for the handling of other high-risk pathogens. In addition, more specific protocols have also been developed for other emerging infectious diseases caused by such pathogens such as highly pathogenic influenza viruses [9] and Middle East Respiratory Syndrome (MERS) coronavirus [10]. These documents also provide templates for guidance as other new infectious diseases are identified.

Laboratories supporting small critical access hospitals or those supporting large acute care facilities therefore need to be prepared to handle specimens that might contain a RG-4 pathogen. This chapter provides simplified information on how to conduct a biological risk assessment, provide measures to mitigate risks, and perform pre-analytical, analytical, and post-analytical processing within a safe environment. In addition, advice is provided on how to expand testing as needed and to sustain readiness of the laboratory when the need for testing specimens that might contain a HCP occurs.

Safety: Risk Assessment and Mitigation

Given the ease of global travel, any facility, regardless of location, may face the need to identify and care for a patient with a dangerous or novel infectious disease. All laboratory workers therefore must be prepared to handle specimens from patients with highly hazardous communicable diseases that may be admitted to their institution [11]. The OSHA general duty clause requires that "employers furnish every employee a workplace that is free from recognized hazards that can cause or are likely to cause death or serious physical harm" [12]. Safety therefore is not a new concept for medical facilities, and procedures should be in place to allow for the safe handling and processing of specimens, no matter what the infectious source.

Recently, the CDC provided a framework for a tiered approach for US medical facilities to provide care for a person under investigation (PUI) for or a patient

Table 6.1 Laboratory resources needed to support the various roles of acute healthcare facilities to manage a patient under investigation for or infected with a high-consequence pathogen[a,b]

Role	Facility needs
Frontline healthcare facilities[c]	Identify and isolate the person under investigation (PUI)
	Training in advanced techniques of PPE
	Training in specimen collection using advanced PPE
	Sufficient PPE to maintain PUI for up to 24 h
	Certified biosafety cabinet (or plastic shield barrier)
	Centrifuge with sealed rotors or safety cups
	Written procedures to safely perform in-house lab testing
	Specimen transport procedures (category A packaging)
Assessment hospitals[d]	Meet all processes for frontline healthcare facilities
	Have minimal laboratory testing capabilities[e]
	Appropriate staffing to operate laboratory 24/7
Treatment centers[f]	Meet all processes for frontline facilities and assessment hospitals
	Have essential laboratory testing capabilities[g]

[a]Prepared from CDC Guidance documents [14–16]
[b]All facilities need to perform a biological risk assessment to identify and mitigate risks
[c]Rapidly identify and isolate patients with relevant exposure history and signs or symptoms, provide laboratory support for up to 24 h of care (to include transport of specimens for confirmation testing), and transport patient to assessment hospital or treatment center if needed
[d]Safely receive and isolate patient, provide laboratory support for up to 5 days (including evaluation and management of alternative diagnoses), and transport patient to a treatment center as needed in consultation with public health officials
[e]Minimal testing capabilities described in guidance documents [7, 11, 21]
[f]Safely receives and provides medical care for a patient with a confirmed high-consequence pathogen to include laboratory support for the duration of the illness
[g]Essential testing capabilities as provided by CDC guidance [7]

infected with EVD [13]. Although this was initially developed with EV in mind, the approach is now being developed around the assessment of any patient with a possible HCP. This tiered approach encompasses designating acute healthcare facilities as either frontline healthcare facilities [14], assessment hospitals [15], or treatment centers [16]. Table 6.1 describes some of the laboratory resources needed to support the various roles in this tiered approach for healthcare facilities.

One major goal of any laboratory to support these various roles for healthcare facilities is to minimize risk to laboratory personnel when handling clinical specimens. To do this, a biological risk assessment is first performed to determine the potential for exposure from sprays, splashes, or aerosols generated during laboratory activities. Although a qualitative assessment is a subjective process that involves professional judgment, the assessment is performed based on the potential of what can happen with assumptions made in the process [7]. The first part of the assessment is to identify the hazards (i.e., activities) that can cause exposure, prioritize the risks, and mitigate the identified risks using engineering controls, administrative controls (work practices), and the use of appropriate personal protective equipment (PPE). Although the utilization of appropriate PPE with training in proper donning and doffing is a critical step for worker safety, the use of a certified biological safety cabinet for primary containment when handling or manipulating patient specimens is also recommended for the laboratory [5, 7, 17]. In addition, laboratory equipment that is used to process specimens should have closed tube processing (i.e., sealed rotor or safety cups for centrifugation), and if open tube processing occurs, the equipment should be manipulated within a biosafety cabinet. The ultimate goal for safety is to protect the laboratorians and environment from contamination while ensuring that an optimal level of care is provided to the patient [18].

Laboratory Testing

Pre-analytical Processes

The pre-analytical processes include the initial screening by triage staff of a PUI, the activation of protocols to isolate the patient during the assessment, the collection of specimens for screening, the transport of specimens to the laboratory, and the activation of a dedicated laboratory if needed. The decision to screen a patient is made in consultation with the relevant local and state health departments with advice as needed from the CDC. Once a decision has been made that laboratory testing is necessary, in-house developed procedures are followed concerning the collection of the specimens in the isolation room (hot zone) as well as the proper procedures to package and transport specimens to the appropriate laboratory for testing [19]. Table 6.2 provides a supply checklist for facilities to safely collect specimens that could possibly contain a HCP.

Prior to the collection of specimens, procedures should be developed to identify best method of collection (line draw, vacutainer, syringe, avoiding butterfly), as well as to identify those who have experience in specimen collection and have been routinely trained in advanced PPE techniques (nurse, laboratorian, phlebotomist, or other medical staff). When collecting a specimen, a partner system is suggested as a means to monitor for a safety breach and to provide a "second pair of hands" to help in the collection and initial processing of the specimens for transport. A recommended step-by-step partner method for specimen collection in the isolation area is provided in Table 6.3.

The initial screening process might include a limited number of specimens such as whole blood (to collect for plasma or serum) or specimens from other body sites such as a respiratory specimens or blood for culture. All facilities should have protocols developed and procedures drilled and exercised on an annual basis to safely collect specimens to evaluate a PUI for a HCP. For instance, guidelines are available to help facilities create appropriate processes to safely collect blood samples as needed [20]. Each step in the collection process should be evaluated by experts in infection control in an effort to limit exposure. This process requires multiple glove changes during the collection, multiple disinfection steps, and triple packaging of specimens within the patient isolation area. In addition, all facilities should have a plan in place to manage other potentially serious medical issues that may develop

Table 6.2 Supply checklist for the collection of specimens from a person under investigation for an infection with a high-consequence pathogen[a–c]

Area	Supplies needed[d]
Isolation (hot zone)	Proper advanced PPE
	Appropriate specimen collection devices
	Appropriate disinfection wipes
	Medical waste container
	Preprinted patient labels with at least 2 identifiers
	Blue or black ink pen[e]
	Small sealable biohazard bags with absorbent material
	Large sealable biohazard bags
Packaging (clean zone)	Insulated category A box system (UN certified)[f]
	Insulated triple packaged system[g]
	Chain of custody paper work[g]
	Appropriate refrigerant
	Appropriate disinfection wipes

[a]Prior permission is required from the local or state public health department to test for a high-risk pathogen
[b]State public health officials should determine the best method to transport specimens to the jurisdictional public health laboratory for confirmation testing
[c]For the collection and transport, follow CDC or public health developed procedures
[d]Check supplies for expiration dates
[e]Used to label specimen collection containers with collector's initials and date/time of collection. Use ink that will not smear when disinfected
[f]If transported by a commercial courier, follow Department of Transportation guidelines for packaging and labeling of these Category A infectious substances
[g]For in-house and local transfer of specimens. Chain of custody may be required for transport from public health laboratory to the CDC

while the PUI is in isolation and awaiting results of confirmation testing. Specific tests might include a complete blood cell count, electrolyte analysis, or specific direct tests for other infectious diseases caused by such pathogens as the influenza viruses, group A *Streptococcus*, and malaria protozoans. For those laboratories that support facilities where these patients might be sent for treatment, a list of essential tests have been described with additional supplemental tests that might be considered (Table 6.4) [7, 21]. Each medical facility needs to define which tests will be available following consultation among the appropriate medical staff and the laboratory administration.

When developing protocols to assess a PUI, facilities should carefully plan what supplies will be needed and the best placement for these supplies so they are readily available when needed. Storage of PPE and specimen collection kits placed near

Table 6.3 Recommended partner method for specimen collection in the isolation area (hot zone)[a,b]

Step 1. Preposition supplies on a clean adjacent table/tray[c]
Step 2. Prepare patient according to specimen collection type(s)
Step 3. Collect specimen(s) following standard procedures and next place on disinfectant wipe open on table/tray
Step 4. Remove top glove, hand sanitize with new disinfectant wipe, and replace top glove
Step 5. Using a new disinfectant wipe, pick up the specimen collection container
Step 6. Wipe each container thoroughly with a new disinfectant wipe to remove any visible blood/specimen
Step 7. Lay specimen containers on a new disinfectant wipe and allow to air-dry
Step 8. Discard disinfectant wipes into the waste container
Step 9. Remove top glove, hand sanitize with a new disinfectant wipe, and replace top glove
Step 10. Pick up the collected specimen using a new disinfectant wipe, and place preprinted label on the container
Step 11. With the help of the partner, place the specimen collection container into a small biohazard bag (secondary container has absorbent material as appropriate)
Step 12. Wipe the outside of the small bag with a new disinfection wipe from bottom to top
Step 13. Carefully fold small bag to expel air and seal
Step 14. With the partners help, place the small biohazard bag(s) containing the collected specimen(s) into a larger biohazard bag (third layer)
Step 15. Repeat steps 10–14 for each specimen collected. All specimens can be placed into one large biohazard bag as space allows
Step 16. Once the specimens are in the large biohazard bag, carefully expel the air and seal
Step 17. With the help of the partner, wipe the outside of the large biohazard bag with a new disinfection wipe
Step 18. The partner not holding the large bag removes top glove, hand sanitizes with a disinfection wipe, and handed the larger bag while holding with a new disinfection wipe
Step 19. Carefully hand the triple packaged specimen(s) to a third person stationed within the clean zone
Step 20. Additional packaging will be done in the clean zone, dependent on where the specimen is to be transported for testing

[a]Following approval, only predesignated staff trained and exercised in the proper PPE and collection procedures will collect specimens

[b]Read out loud the step-by-step checklist when performing the collection process, and observe for any breach in safety

[c]Supplies to include disinfection wipes, specimen collection containers, waste container, preprinted patient labels, ink pen, and small/large biohazard bags

patient isolation areas should not contain supplies with short expiration dates, such as vacutainer tubes or disinfectant wipes. Instead, facilities should consider having supplies made available from the hospital current inventory for immediate availability.

Once a decision has been made to collect specimens and the appropriate specimens have been collected, the next step is to prepare the specimen for transport. Following the transport of the collected specimen(s) to the clean zone, additional packaging will need to be considered prior to transporting the specimen to the laboratory. The level of packaging will be determined by where the specimen is to be

Table 6.4 Other supplemental tests to consider depending on type of illness and travel history

Test	Method[a,b]	Disease
Antimicrobial susceptibility	Manual/automated	Bacterial
Blood culture	Manual/automated	VHF/Resp
Blood type	Manual (agglutination)	VHF
Influenza subtyping[c]	Molecular test[d]	Resp
Group A *Streptococcus*	Manual	Resp
Malaria	Manual/immunological	VHF
MERS	Molecular test[d]	Resp
Respiratory panels	Molecular test	Resp
Troponin	POC test	VHF
Urine	Dipstick manual	VHF
Emerging pathogen[e]	Varies	Varies

Abbreviations: *VHF* unspecified viral hemorrhagic fevers, *Resp* known/unknown respiratory pathogens, *POC* point-of-care, *MERS* Middle East Respiratory Syndrome

[a]The safety risks involved in using an automated or molecular test system need to be considered

[b]Some of these assays involve the use of kits that can be manipulated within a biosafety cabinet.

[c]Includes avian influenza viruses H5 and H7 depending on travel history

[d]Testing for avian influenza and MERS coronavirus is generally performed at the jurisdictional public health laboratory

[e]Rare emerging pathogen detection frequency will require screening to be performed at the CDC using research methods for detection

transported, whether to an adjacent in-unit laboratory, to another on-site laboratory, or to an off-site laboratory (local public health laboratory or federal laboratory). Specimens transported outside of the patient isolation area and through any public area must be triple packaged before transport. These specimens are considered "suspected Category A infectious substances" and therefore must be transported in accordance with OSHA (29 CFR 1910.1030) and DOT (49CFR Part 171–78) guidelines. For safety reasons, this holds true for transport of these high-risk specimens even within the confines of the hospital environment.

Triple packaging consists of a primary receptacle with secondary and outer packaging included. The specimen container used to collect the specimen from the patient is considered the primary receptacle (plastic recommended) and therefore must be sealable and leak-proof. Screw-capped tubes must be secured by adhesive tape and paraffin tape or have a manufactured locking closure. If collecting multiple primary receptacles, each should be placed into separate secondary containers (small biohazard bag). For liquid infectious substances, absorbent material sufficient to absorb all fluids in case of breakage should also be included inside each of the secondary containers. One larger, sealable biohazard bag is then be used as the third layer of packaging.

Triple-packaged specimens that are processed without additional testing within the patient containment unit laboratory can be handed directly to the laboratorian without any further packaging, while those transported outside the patient isolation area are to be packaged following guidance for Category A infectious substance packaging. In addition, a buddy system for specimen transport should be considered with the appropriate security as needed when transporting specimens outside of the patient care area. A log or chain-of-custody form should also be considered for specimen tracking.

Any specimens collected from a PUI that are to be transported outside the facility to the public health laboratory or from the public health laboratory to the CDC should be shipped in UN specification packaging. The shipper must be trained and certified in Division 6.2 packaging (every 2 years) and is legally responsible for complying with all federal regulations for shipment of a Category A infectious substance. Commercial couriers must also meet requirements of the DOT (49CFR part 171–178) to include maintaining sufficient liability and documentation for each shipment. It is important to understand that commercial couriers have restrictions and variations on which Category A infectious substance shipments will be accepted for transport. Most commercial couriers will accept Category A packages that contain a specimen from a PUI for confirmation testing; however, once a patient has been identified as having a known HCP (by culture or by a molecular or serological assay), most commercial couriers will no longer accept these specimens for transport. To address issues for transport off-site using a commercial courier, facilities need to be advised of the complexity in shipping and have plans to address questions that may arise. In lieu of using a commercial courier, federal designation of a public health emergency also allows for law enforcement agents or other designated state or federal officials to transport specimens which have been triple packaged as Category A shipments without the shipper's declaration documentation or specialized training generally required of the transporter.

Facilities also need to be conscious of the regulations pertaining to the handling and shipping of specimens that might contain a select agent pathogen [22]. Current federal law states that specimens obtained from a patient infected with a select agent which are generated during the delivery of patient care are not considered regulated under the select agent regulations if not cultured; thus there are no requirements to document the transfer or destruction of these specimens [23]. However, these specimens are subject to the select agent regulations after acute care of the patient concludes. Further discussion of this issue can be found in the post-analytical section of this chapter describing the storage of excess clinical materials as well.

During the pre-analytical process, there may also be a need for frontline, as well as assessment facilities, to process specimens in-house prior to transfer. These steps might include centrifugation for the collection of plasma or serum, the preparation of a fixed smear for malarial testing, or the extraction of nucleic acid material [24]. A risk assessment should be performed to define where and how these processes can be safely implemented.

Analytical Processes

The analytical processes include those activities involved with the actual testing of the specimens. Having available the appropriate methods and equipment to conduct the laboratory testing are essential parts of this process. Included in this testing process are equipment management plans such as documentation of the original test validation, a continuous validation process during testing, and ongoing calibration criteria as pertaining to reagent testing and validation. As a part of this, all clinical laboratories should have methods in place to provide a sufficient validated laboratory test menu to ensure that the care of the patient is not compromised. Laboratorians also need to be mindful that reference laboratory testing may not be available to handle specimens from these patients and alternative methods for testing need to be considered. Selecting the appropriate methods for testing might also include a combination of manual kit assays such as testing for malaria, pregnancy, or influenza; automated core testing assays such as those for electrolytes, liver function, and coagulation; and to point-of-care (POC) testing devices for multiple activities to include the evaluation for blood gases. The availability of resources and the risk assessment processes will help to determine which of these methods can be utilized safety in the laboratory and what alternative methods are available to provide patient care as needed.

Alternatively, testing for microbial pathogens other than the HCP will generally require kit-based methods. Automated instrument processing such as blood cultures, single-plex and multiplex assays using molecular methods, and identification/susceptibility testing methods need to be evaluated for the biohazard risks. In many instances, manual-based methods can be incorporated to perform the needed test to alleviate the need for processing on an automated instrument where close-tubed testing might not be available. In addition, if lab testing cannot be performed safely, empiric therapies may be considered by the medical care team.

All testing methods require the laboratory to have a quality management plan available to meet Clinical Laboratory Improvement Amendments (CLIA) regulations. These include performing quality control and proficiency testing and documentation that personnel have relevant laboratory education and experience qualification to perform the tests. A process for validation of new methods prior to implementation as well as processes for continued validation of accuracy, precision, and reliability to meet regulatory standards also needs to be considered. Furthermore, instruments will also require an ongoing maintenance plan as required by the manufacturer.

Finally, the ability to have access to validated POC instruments at the site of patient care to perform clinical chemistry and hematological assays, which can be manipulated in a safe environment by competent individuals, is important to meet patient management needs. Numerous POC instruments have been developed that could provide this support (Table 6.5). It is important however to ensure that these instruments are used as approved by the Food and Drug Administration (FDA). For instance, some POC devices that are used to test samples from critically ill patients may be considered off-label use (i.e., glucose meters), requiring that the laboratory establish performance specific for accuracy, sensitivity, specificity, reportable range of test results, reference intervals, and other performance characteristics as required. It is also important to ensure that a quality management program for each instrument be developed to meet all applicable federal and state regulations as well as the standards of the laboratory's accrediting agency and the device manufacturer's instructions. The regulatory standards may differ substantially depending on

Table 6.5 Point-of-care and compact analyzers used to provide laboratory testing in the care of patients known or under investigation for an infection caused by a high-consequence pathogen[a–c]

Instrument	Test Type	CLIA Waived	Measured parameters[e]
Hemochron Jr.® Signature Elite	APTT cuvette	No	APTT
Hemochron Jr.® Signature Elite	PT cuvette	No	PT/INR
Piccolo® Xpress[f]	Liver plus disc	Yes[h]	ALB, ALP, ALT, AMY, AST,GGT, TBIL, TP
Piccolo® Xpress[f]	MetLAC 12 disc	No	ALB, BUN, Ca^{++}, Cl^- CRE, GLU, K^+, Na^+, PHOS, tCO_2, LAC, Mg^{++}
Piccolo® Xpress[f]	MetLYTE plus CRP disc	No	BUN, CK, Cl^-, CRE, GLU, K^+, Na^+, tCO_2, CRP
i-STAT® System[f]	CHEM 8+ cartridge	Yes[i]	Na^+, K^+, Cl^-, AG, iCa^{++}, GLU, BUN, CRE, HCT
i-STAT® System[i]	G3+ cartridge	No	pH, pCO_2, pO_2
Sysmex pocH-100i	pochH-100[i] pack	No	CBC with three-part differential (WBC, RBC, PLT), HGB, HCT
epoc™ blood analysis system	BGEM test card	No	pH, pCO_2, pO_2, Na^+, K^+, Ca^{++}, GLU, LAC, HCT

Abbreviations: *APTT* activated partial thromboplastin, *PT/INR* prothrombin time with international normalized ratio, *ALB* albumin, *ALP* alkaline phosphatase, *ALT* alanine aminotransferase, *AMY* amylase, *AST* aspartate aminotransferase, *GGT* gamma glutamyl transferase, *TBIL* total bilirubin, *TP* total protein, *BUN* blood urea nitrogen, Ca^+ calcium, Cl^- chloride, *CRE* creatinine, *GLU* glucose, K^+ potassium, Na^+ sodium, *PHOS* phosphorus, *LAC* lactate, Mg^+ magnesium, *CK* creatine kinase, *HCT* hematocrit, *HGB* hemoglobin, *CRE* C-reactive protein, *AG* anion gap, pCO_2 partial pressure of carbon dioxide, pO_2 partial pressure of oxygen, *CBC* complete blood cell count, *WBC* white blood cell, *RBC* red blood cell, *PLT* platelet, *CLIA* Clinical Laboratory Improvement Amendments

[a]Controls are run at least daily or more frequently if specified in the manufacturer's instructions when patient testing is performed

[b]A program is available to ensure that each person performing non-waived and waived testing maintains a satisfactory level of competence

[c]An appropriate proficiency testing or alternative assessment program has been established for each assay

[d]Quality control and verification testing are required with each new lot received and if instrument or reagent performance is questioned

[e]Does not include calculated values

[f]These point-of-care instruments have multiple panels/cartridges that can be considered for testing

[g]This instrument performs a "self-check" every time the machine is activated and a test is performed

[h]For testing on whole blood only

[i]For testing on venous samples only

whether a CLIA-waived or non-waived assay is chosen. Frequency of external quality control testing can range from a per reagent lot verification to every 8 h dependent upon the FDA test complexity level, the manufacturers' recommendations, and any applicable accreditation standards. In some cases, external quality control frequency may be reduced by performing a thorough risk assessment of the device and assay and developing an individualized quality control plan (IQCP). Facilities will also need to determine where POC testing is performed (at the bedside, in-unit laboratory, or in-hospital laboratory) and who will perform the testing. Individuals who will be operating the instruments must meet the competency standards as required for each assay. Another advantage of these instruments is the small size and the ability to perform testing within a biosafety cabinet as primary containment for safety. With the proper use of a biosafety cabinet, the potential for exposure to aerosolized highly infectious materials from these POC instruments can be reduced.

Other compact analyzers technically were not developed for POC testing, but are small enough in size to be useful for in-unit or dedicated small lab space testing. The compact size does allow for the placement of these instruments within a biosafety cabinet when testing highly infectious materials. Some instruments use a disc spinning (centrifugation) to perform microfluidic operations and therefore could result in the potential of aerosolization during the testing process [25]. These instruments are not CLIA-waived for all assays, and the testing of patient samples must be validated on-site before they can be used for testing.

Post-analytical Processes

The post-analytical processes include results reporting, reflex testing, waste management, environmental decontamination, storage of excess clinical materials, and an appropriate occupational health plan to monitor employees for potential exposures. The reporting of results becomes complicated when specimens are submitted to multiple laboratories, especially when the reporting involves multiple laboratory information systems (LIS) while maintaining compliance with the Health Insurance Portability and Accountability Act (HIPAA) regulations. Laboratories need to have procedures in place to deal with how the information will be transferred and build in the available LIS test fields to evaluate the reporting processes that will be used. The results reported will also impact what reflex testing might be needed to provide additional information for the care of the patient with the ability to have a rapid turnaround time. This additional testing may require help from not only the jurisdictional public health laboratory but also the submission of specimens to other federal laboratories such as the CDC.

Protocols also need to be developed on how to handle laboratory waste, to include processes for decontamination of specimens and procedures to archive excess clinical materials for follow-up testing (which may be required following experimental drug treatments) or for research in the evaluation of new diseases. Numerous processes have been described for the decontamination of waste that might contain Ebola virus [6, 26, 27]. The Division of Select Agents and Toxins (DSAT) has recently described protocols for the inactivation of select agents [23]. Included is guidance on how to determine non-viability. Although viability testing is no longer considered the standard in all instances, specimen samples that are retained and subsequently identified to contain a select agent pathogen must meet the standards for inactivation that shows the materials contains no viable pathogen-before being retained in a laboratory not approved for the select agent involved.

An additional issue to consider is the decontamination of laboratory equipment after testing samples that may contain a RG-4 pathogen. Manufacturers have provided methods that might be considered, but these range from minimal processing using bleach wipes to incineration of the instrument after utilization [28]. Although studies have shown that 10% bleach at a minimal contact time of 5 minutes is highly effective to inactivate EV and most likely other high-risk pathogens, an internal risk assessment and consultation with manufacturers needs to be considered as protocols are defined to monitor equipment used under these circumstances [29].

Finally, employers whose workers may be at risk of a laboratory-acquired infection are required to have a comprehensive occupational safety and health program to not only anticipate work-related risks but also to describe strategies for protection against these risks [30]. This program needs to be facility specific and includes processes designed so that the healthcare worker will not be subjected to unreasonable burdens such as quarantine in the absence of symptoms. Overall, specifics of working with known or unknown RG-4 pathogens need to be considered on a case-by-case basis.

Sustainability

The Ebola epidemic has engaged laboratory administrators to not only examine their existing capabilities but also to determine laboratory sustainability to respond to an event that may or may not occur in the future. Although frontline hospitals should have programs in place to isolate and assess a PUI for a HCP, the real risk for the diversion of significant funds to be ready for a rare event is for those facilities that will be responsible to provide expanded laboratory support to screen and care for these patients, i.e., assessment hospitals and treatment centers. In addition to an essential list of laboratory tests that will be available to provide care for the HCP patient, the laboratory also needs to define what equipment/supplies are necessary to provide these required tests. The validation of new test protocols and the ability to sustain readiness while adhering to the regulatory requirements to offer testing are costly. These costs include having available and competent staff to support the specialized laboratory testing for an in-unit laboratory, but also the costs for maintenance of accreditation for specialized equipment, equipment depreciation and service contracts, and inventory to keep an adequate supply of reagents available for patient testing (Table 6.6). These are added costs that are necessary to preserve a quality management program that will meet the regulatory requirements of a certified laboratory. Although some governmental support may be available for medical facilities to sustain the capability to provide treatment for patients with HCPs, financial commitment from the facility will also be required. Time will tell how much of an obligation will be necessary for these medical facilities to be in a ready state to care for these patients.

Table 6.6 Major costs to maintain readiness of a laboratory to support the care of a patient infected with a high-consequence pathogen

Cost category	Needs
Training	Personnel have appropriate education and experience
	Regular in-service training on each instrument to maintain competency
	Donning and doffing of PPE
	Working within the containment laboratory
	Competent staffing to operate laboratory 24/7
	Packaging and shipping of Category A substances
Accreditation	All POC tests meet standards for accreditation
	Proficiency testing program participation
	Record maintenance required for accreditation
	Temperature monitoring of equipment and reagent storage
	Patient reporting system
	Test documentation for adverse events
Equipment	Meet all regulatory standards/manufacturers recommendations
	Ongoing equipment assessment
	Service contracts and depreciation
	Preventative maintenance program
Inventory control	Inventory control checklist template
	Adequate storage conditions for reagents
	Monitor shelf life of consumables
	Adequate supplies to provide care upon activation of the laboratory
	Specimen collection devices adequate supply

Abbreviations: *PPE* personal protective equipment, *POC* point-of-care

Conclusions

Laboratorians understand that work in any laboratory, whether classified as high containment or not, is not without risks and that their employer is required to have available the equipment, facilities, and access to specialized training to mitigate these risks. Laboratorians also acknowledge that technology is constantly changing and that adaptation to these changes is necessary. The balance of safety and providing quality results for patient care continues to be a delicate balance for the laboratory. Two future areas that may impact the laboratory overall, but are clearly needed for the high containment labs, include access to specimen collection devices that have the capacity to inactivate pathogens but still allow for the specimen to be acceptable for testing and the development of automated instruments by manufacturers that provide work flow efficiencies that includes close system testing along with specimen tracking. The development of specimen collection devices containing chemicals that can render a pathogen inactive while still stabilizing the specimen for testing has only recently been commercially developed for HIV testing [31, 32]. Additional work needs to be done in this area to expand the commercial availability of these types of collection devices for other applications. Making specimens noninfectious will also enhance the ability to transport and provide the means for in-house, long-term storage of these specimens to evaluate experimental drug applications and for potential future research activities without the regulations of the select agent program. With the development of safer equipment by manufacturers, the ability to test specimens with minimal handling will also reduce exposure opportunities in the laboratory. These and other ongoing changes will help hospitals enhance safety while providing optimal care for patients with infections caused by HCPs.

References

1. Broadhurst MJ, Brooks TJG, Pollock NR. Diagnosis of Ebola virus disease: past, present, and future. Clin Microbio Rev. 2016;29(4):773–93.
2. Polgreen PM, Santibanez S, Koonin LM, Rupp ME, Beekmann SE, Del Rio C. Infectious disease physician assessment of hospital preparedness for Ebola virus disease. Open Forum Infect Dis. 2015;2(3):1–6.
3. Santibanez S, Polgreen PM, Beekmann SE, Rupp ME, Del Rio C. Infectious disease physicians' perceptions about Ebola preparedness early in the US response: a qualitative analysis and lessons for the future. Health Security. 2016;14(5):345–50.
4. Dubov A, Appleton JH, Campbell S. Ebola virus preparedness: emerging viruses and ethics in laboratory medicine. Arch Pathol Lab Med. 2016;140:171–80.
5. Centers for Disease Control and Prevention. CDC guidance on personal protective equipment to be used by Healthcare Workers During Management of Patients with Ebola Virus Disease in U.S. Hospitals, Including Procedures for Putting On (Donning) and Removing (Doffing). 2014. http://www.cdc.gov/vhf/ebola/hcp/procedures-for-ppe.html. Accessed December 6, 2016.
6. Centers for Disease Control and Prevention. Procedures for safe handling and management of Ebola-associated waste. 2014. http://www.cdc.gov/vhf/ebola/healthcare-us/cleaning/handling-waste.html. Accessed March 1, 2018.
7. Centers for Disease Control and Prevention. Guidance for U.S. laboratories for managing and testing routine clinical specimens when there is a concern about Ebola virus disease. 2015. http://www.cdc.gov/vhf/ebola/healthcare-us/laboratories/safe-specimen-management.html. Accessed March 1, 2018.
8. Centers for Disease Control and Prevention. Guidance for collection, transport and submission of specimens for Ebola virus testing. 2015. http://www.cdc.gov/vhf/ebola/healthcare-us/laboratroies/specimens.html. Accessed March 1, 2018.
9. Centers for Disease Control and Prevention. Interim biosafety guidance for all individuals handling clinical specimens or isolates containing 2009-H1N1 Influenza A Virus (Novel H1N1), include Vaccine Strains. 2009. http://www.cdc.gov/h1n1flu/guidelines_labworkers.htm. Accessed March 1, 2018.
10. Centers for Disease Control and Prevention. Interim laboratory biosafety guidelines for handling and processing specimens associated with Middle East Respiratory Syndrome Coronavirus (MERS-CoV). 2016. http://www.cdc.gov/coronavirus/mers/guidelines-lab-biosafety.html. Accessed March 1, 2018.
11. Iwen PC, Smith PW, Hewlett AL, Kratochvil CJ, Lisco SJ, Sullivan JN, et al. Safety considerations in the laboratory testing of specimens suspected or known to contain Ebola virus. Amer. J Clin Pathol. 2015;143(1):4–5.
12. Department of Labor. Occupational Safety and Health Administration, Occupational Health and Safety Act of 1970, Section 5(a)1, Amended 1Jan2004 1970.

13. Centers for Disease Control and Prevention. Interim guidance for U.S. Hospital Preparednesss for Patients Under Investigation (PUIs) or with Confirmed Ebola Virus Disease (EVD): a framework for a tiered approach. 2015. http://www.cdc.gov/vhf/ebola/healthcare-us/preparing/hospitals.html. Accessed March 1, 2018.
14. Centers for Disease Control and Prevention. Hospital preparedness: a tiered approach: interim guidance for preparing frontline healthcare facilities for Patient Under Investigation (PUIs) for Ebola Virus Disease (EVD). 2015. http://www.cdc.gov/vhf/ebola/healthcare-us/preparing/frontline-healthcare-facilities.html. Accessed March 1, 2018.
15. Centers for Disease Control and Prevention. Hospital preparedness: a tiered approach: interim guidance for preparing Ebola assessment hospitals. 2015. http://www.cdc.gov/vhf/ebola/healthcare-us/preparing/assessment-hospitals.html. Accessed March 1, 2018.
16. Centers for Disease Control and Prevention. Hospital preparedness: a tiered approach: interim guidance for preparing Ebola Treatment Centers. 2015. http://www.cdc.gov/vhf/ebola/healthcare-us/preparing/treatment-centers.html. Accessed March 1, 2018.
17. Clinical and Laboratory Standards Institute (CLSI). Protection of laboratory workers from occupationally acquired infections; approved guideline. Wayne: Clinical and Laboratory Standards Institute; 2014.
18. Katz LM, Tobian AA. Ebola virus disease, transmission risk to laboratory personnel, and pretransfusion testing. Transfusion. 2014;54(12):3247–51.
19. Wadman MC, Schwedhem SS, Watson S, Swanhorst J, Gibbs SG, Lowe JJ, et al. Emergency department processes for the evaluation and management of persons under investigation for Ebola virus disease. Ann Emer Med. 2015;66(3):306–14.
20. Clinical and Laboratory Standards Institute. Procedures for the collection of diagnostic blood specimens by venipuncture: approved standard, Sixth Edition, CLSI document H3-A6. In: CLSI, 940 West Valley Road, Suite 1400, editor, Wayne, 19087–1898; 2007.
21. Hill CE, Burd E, Kraft CS, Ryan EL, Duncan A, Winkler AM, et al. Laboratory test support for Ebola patients within a high-containment facility. Lab Med. 2014;45(3):e109–e11.
22. Department of Health and Human Services. 42CFR Part 73, Possession, use, and transfer of select agents and toxins: biennial review. Fed Regist. 2012;77(194):61084–115.
23. Centers for Disease Control and Prevention DHHS. Possession, use, and transfer of select agents and toxins; biennial review of the list of select agents and toxins and enhanced biosafety requirements. Fed Regist. 2017;82(12):6278–94.
24. Centers for Disease Control and Prevention. Malaria Diagnosis (U.S.) – Rapid Diagnostic Test. 2015. http://www.cdc.gov/malaria/diagnosis_treatment/rdt.html. Accessed March 1, 2018.
25. Owen W, Caron J, Genzen J. Liver function testing on the Abaxis Piccolo Xpress: use in Ebola virus disease protocols. Clin Chim Acta. 2015;446:119–27.
26. Jelden KC, Gibbs SG, Smith PW, Hewlett AL, Iwen PC, Schmid KK, et al. Comparison of hospital room surface disinfection using a novel ultraviolet germicidal irradiation (UVGI) generator. J Occup Environ Hyg. 2016;13(9):690–8.
27. Lowe JJ, Hewlett AL, Iwen PC, Smith PW, Gibbs SG. Case study: surrogate testing suggests that chlorine dioxide gas exposure would not inactivate Ebola virus contained in environmental blood contamination. J Occup Environ Hyg. 2015;12:D211–D5.
28. Burnham C, Kwon J, Burd E, Campbell S, Iwen P, Miller MB. Are we there yet? Laboratory preparedness for emerging infectious diseases. Clin Chem. 2017;63(4):1–4.
29. Cooks B, Cutts T, Nikiforuk A, Poliquin P, Court D, Strong J, et al. Evaluating environmental persistence and disinfection of the Ebola virus Makona variant. Viruses. 2015;7(4):1975–86.
30. Ringen K, Landrigan PJ, Stull JO, Duffy R, Melius J, McDiarmid MA. Occupational safety and health protections against Ebola virus disease. Amer J Indust Med. 2015;58:703–14.
31. Kwon E, Minhas V, Phiri T, Wood C, Swindells S, Hunsley BB, et al. Inactivation and viral load quantitation of human immunodeficiency virus in blood collected into Cyto-Chex BCT-blood collection device. J Virol Methods. 2014;196:50–5.
32. Rosenstierne MW, Karlberg H, Bragstad K, Lindegren G, Stoltz ML, Salata C, et al. Rapid bedside inactivation of Ebola virus for safe nucleic acid tests. J Clin Microbiol. 2016;54(10):2521–9.

Staffing

7

Mallory Reimers, Jordan A. Hughes, and Brian T. Garibaldi

Introduction

Staffing a facility for bioemergencies is one of the more complex issues in high containment care. The unique clinical and operational challenges of this environment require the creation of a multidisciplinary team with experience across the care spectrum. At the same time, the need to minimize the number of healthcare workers potentially exposed to highly infectious pathogens requires a model in which team members perform multiple functions that may be outside their normal scope of practice. Healthcare worker and patient safety in this environment is the ultimate measure of a successful staffing model. In the following chapter, we will discuss the choice of model, recruitment and retention of personnel, training, and administrative concerns that must be considered when designing a response to bioemergencies. Each facility is unique, so individual institutions must design their own model based on local factors and considerations.

M. Reimers · J. A. Hughes
Department of Medicine, Johns Hopkins Hospital, Baltimore, MD, USA

B. T. Garibaldi (✉)
Johns Hopkins Biocontainment Unit, Pulmonary and Critical Care,
Johns Hopkins University School of Medicine, Baltimore, MD, USA
e-mail: bgaribal@jhmi.edu

A. Hewlett, A. R. K. Murthy (eds.), *Bioemergency Planning*,
https://doi.org/10.1007/978-3-319-77032-1_7

Staffing Model

Compelled vs. Volunteer Service

The first issue that must be considered in designing a staff model is whether or not staff members will be volunteers (i.e., "self-selectors") or compelled to work in the event of a bioemergency. This decision has both practical and ethical implications for a given facility and is one that is best made at the institutional level. There are advantages and disadvantages of each model. A self-selector team is likely to be highly engaged and enthusiastic, traits that are helpful given the demanding nature of training and clinical work in a high containment environment [1, 2]. It may be possible to recruit volunteer staff members from multiple areas across the institution, which helps to minimize the strain on individual clinical units in the event that the team is activated [2]. However, mobilizing an existing clinical team into service (e.g., an intensive care unit staff) leverages established team unity and takes advantage of an existing multidisciplinary skill set.

A self-selector model may create an environment where individuals are perceived to "opt out" of providing care for patients with certain diseases. In past healthcare crises, the refusal of a subset of providers to care for patients with certain diseases has damaged both institutional morale and the public's perception of the healthcare system [3]. The HIV epidemic of the early 1980s provides a recent example of this potentially controversial issue [4, 5]. On the other hand, mandatory participation might create an environment in which individuals resist participation or refuse to provide care [6]. The decision to employ a self-selector or mandatory model must take into consideration these potential pitfalls. One potential strategy to combat this impression is to remind everyone that the entire institution participates in the care of highly infectious patients. Those who do not directly serve on the unit provide support in other areas of the hospital and help to minimize disruptions in operations for the rest of the facility. Participation in the choice of the staff model by multiple stakeholder groups, as well as a clear institutional message describing the rationale for the decision, will also help to mitigate these issues.

Ultimately the choice of staff model may depend on the scale of the threat at hand; a larger threat may necessitate mobilizing a sizeable team that is beyond the capacity of a volunteer system.

Makeup of the Team

The composition of the care team should reflect the anticipated clinical needs of the unit, including critical care capabilities [7]. The size of the team must also take into account the need for redundancy and the ability to activate quickly [8]. The general principle is to maximize capability while minimizing the number of individuals potentially exposed to a highly infectious pathogen.

Team Leadership

The leadership team should include a physician with experience in infectious diseases and/or critical care as well as a nurse with a strong background in team building and administration. Other key individuals include hospital administrators as well as a nurse educator to assist with preparation and implementation of training [1, 2, 7].

Physician Team

Since most anticipated bioemergencies involve highly hazardous communicable diseases (HHCD) that can produce severe illness, the physician provider team should include individuals with training in both infectious diseases as well as critical care [1, 8, 9]. Procedural support is also essential in a high containment environment. Such support could be provided either by critical care physicians or other providers with experience in procedures such as central line insertion, intubation and airway management, thoracentesis, chest tube insertion, lumbar puncture, and paracentesis. Since high containment units need to be prepared to provide critical care services such as hemodialysis and hemodynamic support, consultants such as nephrologists and cardiologists should be recruited to the team [1]. Depending on local capabilities, surgeons may also be included to provide minor surgical and procedural expertise on the unit. The use of an advanced telecommunications system should be considered, as this allows additional consultants access to the patient, without needing to enter a potentially contaminated space [2].

The care of special populations requires additional consideration. Pediatric providers (Chap. 10) and obstetricians (Chap. 9) may be included based on local capabilities and anticipated need.

Ideally, physicians with a low likelihood of turnover should be recruited to the unit staff, to minimize the need for additional onboarding and training. As a result, medical trainees such as students, residents, and fellows are often not included in bioemergency care teams [8]. The potential ethical implications of such a decision are beyond the scope of this chapter.

Figure 7.1 shows the current composition of the physician team at The Johns Hopkins University Biocontainment Unit, one of the federally designated Regional Ebola and Special Pathogens Treatment Centers [10].

Nursing Team

Similar to the physician providers, the nursing team should reflect the anticipated clinical needs of the unit. As a result, it is important to recruit as many nurses as possible with critical care or emergency department experience to provide care for severely ill patients [11, 12]. While it may not be possible to field an entire nursing team with critical care expertise, there needs to be a core group of nurses with such experience so that each clinical shift can have a critical care provider at the bedside

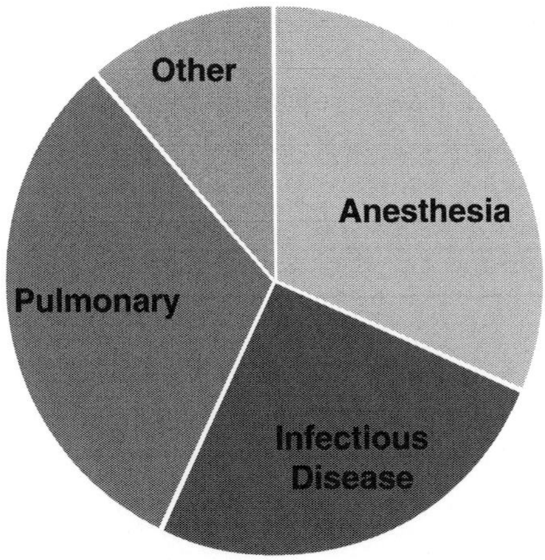

Fig. 7.1 Clinician staff composition of The Johns Hopkins Biocontainment Unit (n = 35 providers)

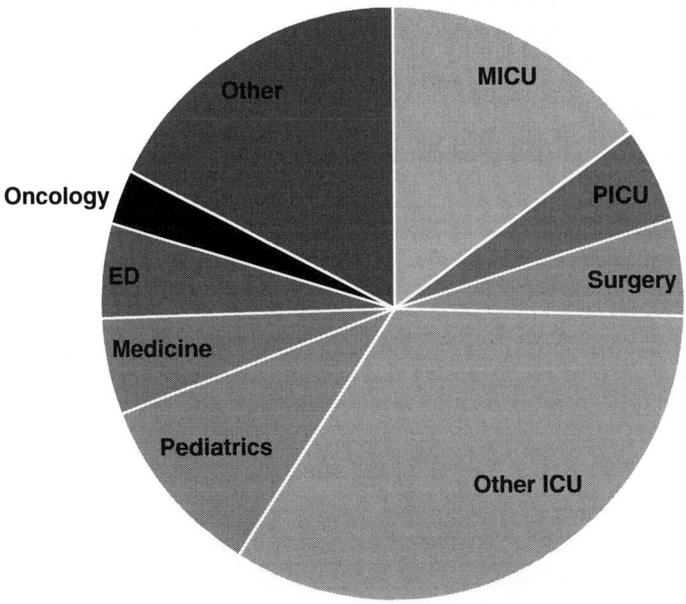

Fig. 7.2 Nurse staff composition of The Johns Hopkins Biocontainment Unit (n = 39; ED = Emergency Department; PICU = Pediatric Intensive Care Unit; MICU = Medical Intensive Care Unit)

if needed [2]. Depending on local needs, the team may include pediatric and obstetric nurses. It is also helpful to recruit nurses with experience in hemodialysis to support the clinical needs of severely ill patients.

Figure 7.2 shows the current composition of The Johns Hopkins University Biocontainment Unit nursing team.

Infection Control Practitioners

The safety of patients and healthcare workers is of the utmost importance in bioemergencies. Infection preventionists (IPs) and/or biosafety officers are critical to the design and successful implementation of care protocols [1, 2, 8, 13]. During activation, they can provide direct observation during clinical care as well as assistance during high-risk activities such as doffing. The number of IPs that are needed depends in part on the size of the clinical unit, since additional patient beds might require increased direct observation by infection control staff.

Additional Staff

Additional staff should be included on the care team based on anticipated service needs, as well as local restrictions in the activities that physicians and nurses are able to perform [2]. For example, local regulations may require that only certified x-ray technologists are able to operate portable imaging devices. The following specialties are routinely recruited to high containment care teams: respiratory therapists, laboratory technologists, X-ray technicians, and dialysis nurses [11]. Depending on local capabilities, the team might include surgical technicians and other operating room staff. Some centers might also recruit perfusionists and specialized cardiovascular nurses in the event that extracorporeal membrane oxygenation (ECMO) is needed for patients with acute respiratory failure from viral infections such as the Middle East respiratory syndrome (MERS) [14, 15]. In order to minimize the number of individuals that enter the unit, routine tasks that are normally performed by patient care technicians, environmental services staff, and other ancillary staff should be handled by unit staff such as nurses and physicians wherever possible.

Employee Health Screening and Monitoring

It is important that all staff are properly screened before being allowed to practice in a high containment environment. This will ensure that staff are capable of performing anticipated duties as safely as possible. This screening process will vary by institution, but there are some components that should be included at all centers. For example, since many high containment pathogens require respiratory protective equipment such as powered air purifying respirators (PAPRs) or N95 masks, providers must pass institutional occupational health requirements to wear such devices. Providers should also undergo routine fitness for duty evaluations commensurate with their institutional policies [1, 8]. Providers need to demonstrate a commitment to a culture of safety [13], both in their daily positions in the hospital and in their participation in containment care activities. This includes participation in mandatory training activities and attention to teamwork and accountability in practice.

Containment care providers should be up to date on appropriate vaccinations in accordance with current Advisory Council on Immunization Policy (ACIP) guidelines for healthcare workers [16]. Most units do not require vaccination against smallpox in the absence of a credible threat or known outbreak of this disease, but it might be reasonable to screen providers beforehand for contraindications to receiving the smallpox vaccine in the event of a documented case [1, 8]. Staff members should also be routinely screened for tuberculosis (TB) since units may be called upon to provide care for resistant cases of TB [8].

Once a provider team is activated, there needs to be a system in place for monitoring staff members for evidence of possible active disease [17]. Monitoring requirements will vary based on the pathogen of interest so facilities should have a plan in place that is flexible enough to meet the needs of candidate diseases. At many institutions, occupational health can facilitate monitoring of staff [2]. Technological aids such as mobile and web-based applications can make the process easier, particularly when monitoring large numbers of individuals [18].

Administrative Logistics

Staffing of the Patient Care Facility During Activation

Ensuring adequate staffing in the event of a bioemergency is crucial to effective operations. When determining staffing requirements for facilities, planning for redundancies and back-up support is key to prepare for unforeseen circumstances, such as travel, illness, or refusal to work [8]. Staffing models and ratios may vary by facility and by specific disease. The Johns Hopkins Biocontainment Unit's (BCU) staff model during activation for a viral hemorrhagic fever is highlighted in Table 7.1.

In this model, nurse roles include charge, bedside, in-room buddy, autoclave operator, tasker, and donning/doffing assistant. The number of in-room nurses may change based on the pathogen at hand. Hospital infection control officers are present to supervise infection control practices, provide step-by-step instructions for the donning and doffing process, and observe in-room providers during clinical care [2]. The nurse manager is stationed outside of the unit in the incident command center to provide oversight and leadership. A supply clerk is present during the day hours to gather necessary supplies and to accept medication, equipment, or additional supplies that are delivered to the unit.

Table 7.1 Sample staffing model during activation

Staff type	# of staff per 12-hour shift
Physician	1
Nurse	6 during day shift
	5 during night shift
Infection control officers	2–3
Nurse manager	1
Supply clerk	1 during day shift only

A call system must be developed to activate the unit in a timely fashion. In the Hopkins system, one physician is always on call to staff the unit within 4 h of activation. Once providers receive notification of activation, there needs to be a clear system for assembling the remainder of the care team. An online scheduling system facilitates this process by allowing physicians to schedule a minimum number of shifts over a predetermined period of time. Similar to physician scheduling, an online system allows self-selector nurses to populate a 6-week schedule in advance of activation. This schedule mirrors their regular clinical schedules to ensure that there are always BCU self-selector nurses working in the hospital in the event of activation. Unlike physician providers, nurses are exclusively assigned to the BCU and do not perform shifts on their regular units during times of activation [2].

Minimizing Disruption to the Healthcare Facility

One of the primary goals in designing a biocontainment staffing strategy is creating a model that minimizes the disruption to the rest of the healthcare facility. A number of actions can be taken to minimize the impact when a unit is activated in a self-selector staffing model:

1. Negotiate with nursing and physician leadership to support and provide backfill for those who choose to serve on the unit.

   At The Johns Hopkins Hospital, the leadership of the biocontainment unit engaged the Division Directors of the self-selected physicians. The Division Directors agreed to provide backfill support to minimize impact on the rest of the hospital [2]. In addition to physician leadership, nursing leadership should be approached to backfill nursing positions on their regular units [19].
2. Create limitations on the number of nurses and staff from the same unit to serve when activated.

   In a volunteer system, it is recommended that limits are placed on the number of nurses from the same unit who serve during an activation event. At The Johns Hopkins Hospital, only four nurses from the same clinical unit work during a 3-week period to limit the shortage of staff on their home clinical units [2]. In a compelled service model, these considerations do not apply as staff from a single clinical group, often the ICU, serve on the biocontainment unit as part of their normal clinical duties. Staff rotate between shifts on the ICU and biocontainment unit, meaning there is less impact to the rest of the hospital, but potentially significant impact to that clinical unit.

Staff Compensation and Finances

When creating the staffing model of a biocontainment unit, staffing costs must be identified for both standby and activation modes. For care teams to be successful during activation, it is crucial that staff are trained on a regular basis to maintain skills and build comradery. Most facilities pay regular wages for any hours spent on preparedness or training activities to retain, engage, and motivate staff members. Not only does this reward staff for their commitment to the team, but it also makes it financially feasible for them to participate in activities outside of their regular work hours.

While some facilities may choose to institute on-call pay for clinical providers during activation, a number of facilities have instituted regular pay for the time worked during activation [19]. This should also extend to events when the unit is not activated such as initial orientation, skills training sessions, drill activities, and staff meetings.

Beyond paying regular wages for the time spent on biocontainment unit activities, creative strategies have also been identified to provide compensation for salaried clinical providers' time spent preparing and training. One example is creating a discretionary account for self-selected physicians to cover scholarly and training activities such as conferences, travel, or external training sessions. Providers must meet basic requirements of participation in the unit, such as participating in drills, attending quarterly training sessions, and agreeing to be on call as needed, to receive the stipend. This method allows a unit to reward providers for their efforts and ensures the provider team is training regularly despite their busy schedules.

Communications

Internal and external communications are necessary to educate, recruit, and motivate staff. When a BCU is opened, communications should be sent to all hospital staff – including e-mail, town hall meetings, departmental meetings, and internal newsletters or publications [2, 19]. The marketing and communications department should be directly involved in these communication efforts, as well as in the event of an activation, to disseminate information to the organization and to the media as needed.

An important way to maintain interest in the activities of the BCU when on standby is to utilize internal communications to the staffing team, as well as to the healthcare facility. At The Johns Hopkins Hospital, the biocontainment unit maintains a monthly blog that shares activities of the unit and care team, including training, drills, speaker sessions, and research activities. The unit also regularly updates a public website for the biocontainment unit to provide news updates, including accomplishments of the staff both inside and outside of the biocontainment unit. Not only does this serve as a way to engage and recognize staff, but it also demonstrates the contributions of the biocontainment unit to the greater community even when the unit is not activated.

In the event the unit is activated, strong communication throughout the care team is critical for staff and patient safety. One recommendation is to utilize a telecommunication system, which allows providers and family members to interact with patients and staff remotely. This enables patients to spend time with loved ones, allows consultative services to occur without entering contaminated areas, and allows staff to communicate and watch each other's actions on the unit hands-free [2].

Staff Engagement

One of the most difficult challenges in maintaining preparedness for a bioemergency is keeping staff engaged during times of unit inactivity. In addition to regular interdisciplinary training sessions (see Chap. 13), it is important to encourage shared problem solving and planning [20]. For example, a continuous open dialogue around policy and protocol development allows staff to feel that their feedback is valued and creates a sense of empowerment [19]. Recognizing staff for their service, both among the team and in the surrounding community, can also foster a strong sense of team unity and accomplishment.

Inviting staff to participate in academic activities related to HHCD is another way to stimulate excitement and engagement. For example, at The Johns Hopkins Hospital, BCU staff members are encouraged to present at regional and national meetings, coauthor manuscripts, attend training sessions at other facilities, and participate in professional development activities such as leadership or educational courses. Quarterly staff meetings also provide opportunities to educate staff about the latest developments in HHCD and containment care.

Future Directions

The formation of dedicated teams to provide care for patients with HHCD has raised a number of important questions about staffing models. For example, the issue of volunteer versus compelled service in the context of HHCD has rekindled previous discussions about the ethical obligations of healthcare providers. The development of advanced technologies for both diagnosis and prognostication may further inform these debates and provide fertile ground for discussing the ethical, legal, and social implications of such advances on healthcare delivery in general. For example, if emerging genomic technologies provide information about staff susceptibility to a specific disease, this might change our current perspective on who is best able to serve in a bioemergency. The current design of staffing models, including the number of providers required to adequately staff a unit, can also be informed by the application of human factors engineering principles, using the data gathered from past and future bioemergency responses.

Conclusions

Staffing a team for bioemergencies is one of the more complex aspects of providing care for patients infected with HHCDs. Staffing models are not one size fits all and must be tailored to meet the needs of facilities and specific crises. Organizations must consider their strengths when organizing a care team. This will allow decisions to be made regarding volunteer versus mandatory service, composition of the team, scheduling of shifts, and training. Recruitment and retention of staff committed to a culture of safety is critical to success, which is measured not only by patient outcome but by healthcare worker and community safety. Future research and additional bioemergency responses will continue to inform the most appropriate ways to structure staffing models that take into account relevant safety, efficacy, and ethical issues.

References

1. Bannister B, Puro V, Fusco FM, Heptonstall J, Ippolito G. Framework for the design and operation of high-level isolation units: consensus of the European Network of Infectious Diseases. Lancet Infect Dis. 2009;9:45–56.
2. Garibaldi BT, Kelen GD, Brower RG, Bova G, et al. The creation of a biocontainment unit at a Tertiary Care Hospital: The Johns Hopkins Medicine Experience. Ann Am Thorac Soc. 2016;13:600–8.
3. Sokol DK. Virulent epidemics and scope of healthcare workers' duty of care. Emerg Infect Dis. 2006;12:4.
4. Link RN, Feingold AR, Charap MH, Freeman K, Shelov SP. Concerns of medical and pediatric house officers about acquiring AIDS from their patients. Am J Public Health. 1988;78:455–9.
5. Freedman B. Is there a duty to provide medical care to HIV-infectious patients? Facts, fallacies, fairness, and the future. Can Fam Physician. 1990;36:479–82.
6. Narasimhulu DM, Edwards V, Chazotte C, Bhatt D, Weedon J, Minkoff H. Healthcare workers' attitudes toward patients with Ebola virus disease in the United States. Open Forum Infect Dis. 2016;3:ofv192.
7. Decker BK, Sevransky JE, Barrett K, Davey RT, Chertow DS. Preparing for critical care services to patients with Ebola. Ann Intern Med. 2014;161:831–2.
8. Smith PW, Anderson AO, Christopher GW, Cieslak TJ, et al. Designing a biocontainment unit to care for patients with serious communicable diseases: a consensus statement. Biosecur Bioterror. 2006;4:351–65.
9. Kortepeter MG, Kwon EH, Hewlett AL, Smith PW, Cieslak TJ. Containment care units for managing patients with highly hazardous infectious diseases: a concept whose time has come. J Infect Dis. 2016;214:S137–41.
10. HHS. HHS selects nine regional Ebola and other special pathogen treatment centers. 2015. Available from: http://www.hhs.gov/about/news/2015/06/12/hhs-selects-nine-regional-ebola-and-other-special-pathogen-treatment-centers.html.
11. Torabi-Parizi P, Davey RT Jr, Suffredini AF, Chertow DS. Ethical and practical considerations in providing critical care to patients with Ebola virus disease. Chest. 2015;147:1460–6.
12. Johnson SS, Barranta N, Chertow D. Ebola at the National Institutes of Health: perspectives from critical care nurses. AACN Adv Crit Care. 2015;26:6.
13. Hewlett AL, Varkey JB, Smith PW, Ribner BS. Ebola virus disease: preparedness and infection control lessons learned from two biocontainment units. Curr Opin Infect Dis. 2015;28:343–8.
14. Al-Dorzi HM, Aldawood AS, Khan R, Baharoon S, Alchin JD, Matroud AA, Al Johany SM, Balkhy HH, Arabi YM. The critical care response to a hospital outbreak of Middle East respiratory syndrome coronavirus (MERS-CoV) infection: an observational study. Ann Intensive Care. 2016;6:101.
15. Choi WS, Kang C-I, Kim Y, Choi J-P, The Korean Society of Infectious D, et al. Clinical presentation and outcomes of Middle East respiratory syndrome in the Republic of Korea. Infect Chemother. 2016;48:118–26.
16. Centers for Disease Control and Prevention (CDC). Immunization of health-care personnel: recommendations of the Advisory Committee on Immunization Practices (ACIP). 2011 [cited 24 Feb 2017]. Available from: https://www.cdc.gov/mmwr/preview/mmwrhtml/rr6007a1.htm.

17. Fink D, Cropley I, Jacobs M, Mepham S. Febrile illness in healthcare workers caring for Ebola virus disease patients in a high-resource setting. Euro Surveill. 2017;22
18. Dishneau D. App aids monitoring of West Africa travelers for Ebola. Baltimore Sun; 2015.
19. Lenaghan PA, Schwedhelm M. Nebraska biocontainment unit design and operations. J Nurs Adm. 2015;45:4.
20. Schwedhelm S, Beam EL, Morris RD, Sebastian JG. Reflections on interprofessional team-based clinical care in the ebola epidemic: the Nebraska Medicine experience. Nurs Outlook. 2015;63:27–9.

Transportation of Patients in a Bioemergency

8

Lekshmi Kumar and Alexander P. Isakov

The 2014–2016 Ebola outbreak increased awareness worldwide of the burden of infectious diseases. Although noncommunicable diseases are the leading cause of morbidity and mortality in most developed nations, infectious diseases remain a major public health concern in the United States and around the world. With globalization and travel, there is a heightened need for preparedness. Systems and processes need to be in place to not just recognize and treat affected individuals but transport them safely with minimal risk of spread.

Prevention of transmission is paramount. Environmental and administrative controls, together with work practices and personal protective equipment must be implemented to prevent direct person-to-person spread via contact with infectious body fluids or droplets and also by indirect spread through fomites. In this chapter we provide a framework for transportation of patients in both the out-of-hospital and hospital settings. Preparedness planning and infection control strategies for each illness need to account for routes of transmission and risk of exposure.

Out-of-Hospital Transport

Healthcare and relief workers traveling to the epicenter of epidemics to provide care is increasingly commonplace. With this there is an increased need to repatriate ill workers and to be vigilant for returning travelers who develop signs and symptoms of illness. Systems and processes need to be in place to recognize signs and symptoms of illness and to manage patients with highly hazardous communicable

L. Kumar (✉) · A. P. Isakov
Section of Prehospital and Disaster Medicine, Department of Emergency Medicine, Emory University School of Medicine, Atlanta, GA, USA
e-mail: lekshmi.kumar@emory.edu

A. Hewlett, A. R. K. Murthy (eds.), *Bioemergency Planning*,
https://doi.org/10.1007/978-3-319-77032-1_8

diseases (HHCD) in the out-of-hospital setting, whether that be a planned intercontinental critical care transport, a domestic interfacility transport, or a local emergency medical services (EMS) response to a medical emergency. Ideally dedicated teams, educated about HHCDs and trained in fastidious implementation of infection control practices, would be available for the planned transport of these patients, but emergency medical services responders will also need to be sufficiently knowledgeable and trained to manage a patient with a HHCD, should the patient's condition preclude waiting for a dedicated team [1]. Outlined are the descriptions of practices that will need to be considered.

Hierarchy of Controls

A hierarchy of controls is used to protect healthcare workers, patients, and others from exposure to infectious bodily fluids, droplets, and aerosols [2]. The hierarchy ranks interventions based on their effectiveness in reducing the likelihood of exposure. In order of preference, the hierarchy describes (1) elimination of potential exposures, (2) engineering/environmental controls, (3) administrative controls/ work practices, and (4) safety/personal protective equipment.

Elimination of Potential Exposure

Eliminating exposure for EMS personnel is a challenge, but plausible in certain contexts. Patients that are known to have a HHCD or are highly suspected of having one, when possible, should preferentially be transported only by personnel and agencies that have the requisite education and training, policies and procedures, demonstrated competencies, and qualified supervision to manage and transport the patient safely. In communities where these capabilities exist, and where there is need for a planned transport of a patient with a HHCD, untrained personnel can avoid exposure. A ready example of a planned transport is an interfacility transport of a patient from one hospital to another (e.g., from a community hospital to a specialty center). Another example of a planned transport is a traveler recently returned from a country with widespread transmission of a HHCD who is being actively monitored by the public health authority for fever and other signs of illness. When it is determined that the traveler has fallen ill and is in need of a medical assessment, qualified teams can be designated to transport the patient, avoiding exposure for others.

When patients access healthcare by dialing 911, it is difficult for emergency responders to eliminate the possibility of exposure. However, call center screening for travel history and signs and symptoms of illness that raise concern about a HHCD can help by alerting the responders to the risk, allowing them to rightsize the response team and eliminate potential exposure for other personnel [3].

Engineering and Environmental Controls

These rank second on the hierarchy of controls, as the implementation of environmental controls decreases the likelihood of exposure without requiring active

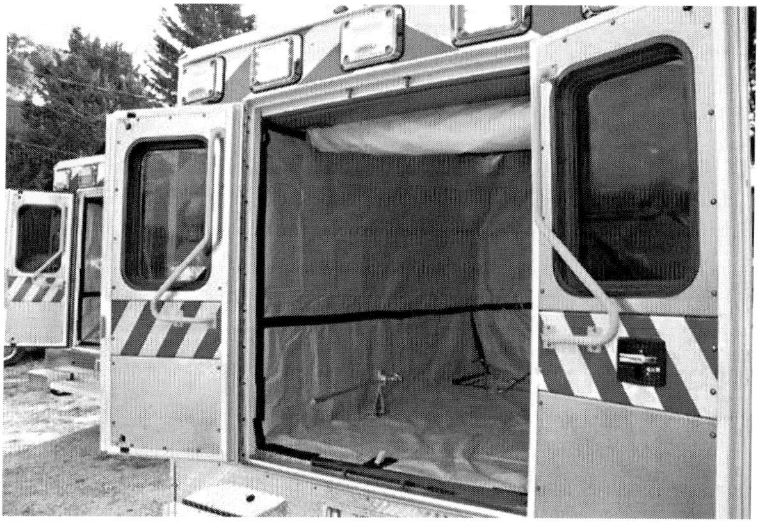

Fig. 8.1 Ambulance with impervious barrier drapes applied as an environmental control. (Photo courtesy of Alex Isakov)

healthcare worker interaction. Environmental controls aim to manage the hazard such that it does not come in contact with the healthcare worker or other personnel. An example of implementation of environmental controls for out-of-hospital management and transport of a patient with a HHCD is modification and preparation of the ambulance or transport vehicle. For example, when transporting a patient confirmed or suspected of having a HHCD, the driver compartment should be isolated from the patient compartment, so that the driver compartment can always be considered clean. In case of transport of patients that require airborne precautions or those requiring aerosol-producing procedures, a positive-pressure environment should be created in the driver compartment using the ventilation system [4]. The ventilation system in the driver compartment should be set in non-recirculating mode with the fan on high. The ventilation system in the back of the ambulance will preferentially also not recirculate air, and the exhaust fan should also be set on high [5]. This should decrease the likelihood of exposure to an infectious aerosol in the driver compartment and maintains appropriate air exchange in the patient compartment.

Depending on the type of vehicle used for transport, the interior needs to be prepared to minimize exposure of environmental surfaces and equipment as well as facilitate decontamination and disinfection following the mission. Various methods have been used to envelop the interior of the patient compartment with impervious barriers to protect against contamination of surfaces [5] (Fig. 8.1). This is especially important for patients who pose a high risk for sharing infectious bodily fluids through active bleeding, vomiting, or diarrhea. The stretcher can be protected with an impervious sheet, and essential medical equipment can be placed in a clear plastic bag [6].

Patients may also be asked to wear a disposable undergarment to capture diarrhea and may be asked to wear a coverall to protect the healthcare worker from draining wounds, or contaminated clothing. If a patient is unable to comply, impervious sheets may be used to envelop the patient during transport. A patient isolation unit may be employed as an environmental control. This has been described for long fixed-wing transports. A portable isolation unit may also be employed by ground or rotor wing air ambulances. Agencies electing to use portable isolation units will need to consider operating procedures for patient management and the unit's decontamination and disinfection or final disposition.

Administrative Controls

Administrative controls are policies and work practices that the healthcare worker implements to avoid exposure and to prevent exposure of others. These rank third in the hierarchy of controls because they require consistent application by healthcare workers and supervisors. There are many examples of policies and work practices implemented to protect the healthcare workers whose scope of work requires management and transport of patients with serious communicable diseases. The application of screening questions to identify patients with fever and other signs and symptoms of illness, like cough, rash, vomiting, or diarrhea, can alert the healthcare worker to the risk of exposure prior to contact [3]. Healthcare workers must fastidiously apply standard precautions with every patient contact, which includes strict adherence to hand hygiene, the use of exam gloves, and the application of other protective equipment to protect the skin and mucous membranes from exposure to bodily fluids. Standard precautions also address the proper cleaning and disinfection of medical equipment and environmental surfaces and the proper use of sharps. In addition to standard precautions, transmission-based precautions may also be required when standard precautions alone do not adequately protect the healthcare worker from the contagion.

Other examples of work practices include limiting the number of healthcare workers making patient contact, prohibiting healthcare worker reentry into the driver compartment of the ambulance after making patient contact, preventing unprotected contact with the patient, and the utilization of trained observers and checklists for the donning and doffing of PPE. Standard clinical care guidelines may need to be modified for transport to enhance safety by avoiding invasive and aerosol-producing procedures when possible and decreasing exposure to sharps in a moving vehicle. Patients may be administered anti-nausea or antidiarrheal medications to decrease the likelihood of emesis or diarrhea. Procedures must be in place for managing breaches of PPE and inadvertent exposure to bodily fluids, as well as for immediate consultation with medical control for decision support. Procedures should also be in place to inform how the patient will be transferred out of or into a hospital. The patient should be transported to the designated location via the most direct path in a manner that limits exposure to unprotected staff, patients, and visitors. Hospital or facility security should be in place to secure the route and guide the transport personnel to the designated unit [7]. A post transport medical surveillance program should be implemented for the care team to ensure early recognition of signs of illness [3].

Safety Equipment and PPE

Safety equipment and PPE ranks last in the hierarchy of controls because it serves as the last line of defense against exposure to infectious bodily fluids, when other controls cannot avoid exposure. Selection of PPE should be based on standard- and transmission-based precautions and in accordance with CDC guidelines. PPE selection should also accommodate the condition of the patient, the anticipated mission requirements, and the work environment [6].

Application of PPE in adherence with standard precautions should include exam gloves during any patient contact and goggles/face shield and simple mask for any airway procedures (intubation, suctioning), with addition of a gown for any situations likely to generate splash/liquid exposures [8]. In cases of large draining wounds or diseases requiring contact precautions, a disposable fluid-resistant gown that extends to at least mid-calf or disposable fluid-resistant coveralls should be used along with disposable gloves in addition to standard precautions. A disposable surgical facemask should be used at all times for droplet precautions, and eye protection may also be advised. In case of airborne illnesses, respiratory protection against inhalation of aerosols is key. PPE includes a disposable National Institute for Occupational Safety and Health (NIOSH)-approved, fit-tested N95 respirator or powered air-purifying respirator (PAPR) with full hood and high-efficiency particulate air (HEPA) filter. PAPRs should be considered for employees that cannot safely fit test on N95 masks due to facial hair, facial structure, etc. [9]. In case of highly pathogenic organisms like EVD, Marburg virus, or Lassa fever, PPE is based on extent of symptoms and presence of active emesis, diarrhea, or bleeding [10].

On prolonged missions, powered air-purifying respirators may be more comfortable when airborne precautions are required. The use of a hooded PAPR may also help avoid other challenges such as fogging of eyewear and risk of inadvertently touching the face. Splash risk with bodily fluids is also decreased [11]. Consider work rest cycles for personnel wearing PPE. Personnel should be competent with donning and doffing equipment. Donning and doffing should be performed under the supervision of a trained observer. The CDC and ASPR have checklists available for donning and doffing procedures as a guideline as well as training resources [3, 11].

Education and Training

As a matter of policy and a commitment to safe practice, paramedics, emergency medical technicians, flight nurses, EMS physicians, and other out-of-hospital healthcare workers need to be educated about infectious pathogens that they may become exposed to in the workplace. They should receive education on signs and symptoms of illness, modes of transmission, incubation periods, available treatments and vaccines, and general management of the patient. Most importantly they must be educated to interrupt transmission with emphasis on standard- and transmission-based infection control practices (Fig. 8.2) [5]. This education is important to mitigate any fears or apprehensions and facilitate the delivery of safe and effective care.

- Introduction and overview of transport of patients with serious communicable disease
  - Education and training
  - Equipment
  - Concept of operations
- Tenets of infection control
  - Standard precautions
    - Hand hygiene
    - PPE
    - Patient care equipment
    - Environmental controls
    - Injury prevention
  - Transmission-based precautions (contact, droplet, aerosol)
    - PPE
    - Patient care equipment
    - Patient placement
    - Categorization of common pathogens
- Education about serious communicable pathogens
  - Epidemiology of illness
  - Microbiology of pathogen
  - Methods of acquisition/transmission
  - Natural disease course
    - Incubation
    - Signs and symptoms
    - Transmission
    - Recovery
  - Preventing transmission/infection control
  - Treatment
  - Vaccine/prophylaxis
- Operational planning and procedures
  - Clinical care guidelines
  - Crew composition and roles
  - Vehicle preparation
  - Special equipment
  - PPE
    - Selection
    - Donning
    - Doffing
  - Decontamination and disinfection procedures
  - Waste management
  - Partnership with receiving facilities
  - Postmission surveillance

Fig. 8.2 Education and training

Healthcare workers are also trained in use of personal protective ensembles. Developing and maintaining a high level of competency with the use of PPE is vital for workforce safety. This should also include fit testing per Occupational Safety and Health Administration (OSHA) Respiratory Protection Standard (29 CFR 1910.134) [12]. Initial training should be followed up with periodic refreshers and exercises prior to a mission.

Additional training on communications, patient care during transport, infection control practices, PPE selection, donning/doffing PPE, and decontamination is also needed [7]. After initial instruction, team medic competency-based training must be evaluated, with special attention to the proper donning and doffing of a variety of personal protective ensembles in the presence of a trained observer.

Special Considerations

Stakeholders

Key stakeholders must be identified early and depending on the case and jurisdiction may include federal, state, and local governments, state or local department of health, and emergency management authorities, state and local EMS and law enforcement agencies, healthcare systems, unions, and others. Relationship building and coordination among these agencies is vital, and coordinated planning and training helps ensure a smooth transport of the patient.

State and local authorities should be involved in facilitating transport and ensuring proper authorities are available to respond to any issues related to the route during transport (traffic, weather-related events). In case of transport involving an airport, airport authorities should be included in mission planning. Multidisciplinary coordination is key for a safe transport. Relationships should be established and time taken to develop and exercise SOPs. Training exercises will provide an opportunity to execute a step-by-step plan and provide the various agencies an opportunity to examine the interface of their respective roles and responsibilities.

Federal authorities also participate in planning and coordination for patient transport and have resources and capabilities which include movement of patients by air ambulance. These resources are largely coordinated by the Department of Health and Human Services, through its Office of the Assistant Secretary for Preparedness and Response. The Centers for Disease Control and Prevention and NIOSH provide guidelines that can be adopted by state and local agencies that will facilitate safe management and transport of patients with HHCDs [7].

Clinical Care Guidelines

Plans for resuscitation and/or active treatment during transport must be considered in case of clinical deterioration and/or death. The transport team should understand which interventions and procedures might be anticipated and which will not be considered during the transport (e.g., cardiac arrest resuscitation, intubation, or other invasive procedures) [13]. Plans should consider patient condition, required devices and medication needs, types of PPE necessary, and length of transport time [7]. Consider involving ethics and infectious diseases experts in the planning and discussion.

Ensure that capabilities and protocols exist for transporting pediatric patients, with details for how to handle those with special healthcare needs. Include plans for patients with functional or access needs (e.g., hearing, vision, limited mobility), device dependence, and limited English proficiency. Consider the developmental stage of the patient, especially with pediatric patients, when addressing fears associated with PPE, fears of not having family members present, and an understanding of the transport process [14]. Advance preparation with tabletop exercises and mock drills will help minimize staff apprehension and will assist in implementing timely infection control precautions while maintaining care standards.

The service medical director should be involved in the development of all these guidelines. EMS medical directors ensure quality patient care, with responsibilities including the ongoing design, operation, evaluation, and revision of the EMS system from initial patient access to final patient care destination, the development of medical policies and procedures, and ensuring that patient care activities performed by EMS providers are appropriate and within their scope of practice [15]. The EMS medical director will be actively involved in planning/preparation and available for consultation during interfacility transport.

Communication

Communications can be challenging for the transport team, given the need for personal protective equipment and concern about contaminating equipment. Communications can be facilitated by hands-free radios or devices, which are worn inside the protective ensemble, to prevent exposure to bodily fluids. When communications are not encrypted, the transport team should be careful to protect privileged health information. Transport team supervisory personnel should conduct the majority of the communication with external agencies like police, security, receiving facility, etc. to allow the clinical team to focus on patient care.

Anticipating and preparing for public interest and media attention is key to educating the community and maintaining their confidence. Risk communications should be incorporated into the transport plan. Messaging should be proactive and short, using plain language while adhering to risk communication principles. Media relations and communications officers with experience in emergency risk communication should be identified in advance to manage public interest and media relations. They can also be used to provide communications guidance to the individuals or agencies involved in the transport [16].

Post Mission

Once the transport is completed, the providers involved should be debriefed and post mission surveillance initiated. Appropriate public health, emergency management, and public safety authorities need to be informed. The receiving facility should continue communications with the transporting agency regarding any further positive diagnostic tests on the patient that may impact transport team surveillance or prophylaxis.

Decontamination and Disinfection

The ambulance is decontaminated and disinfected and the transport team doffs their PPE [3] under supervision of qualified and trained personnel. Significant risk for inadvertent exposure occurs especially during doffing potentially contaminated PPE [17]. The interior of the ambulance, the stretcher, and any exposed equipment are disinfected with an Environmental Protection Agency-registered hospital-grade disinfectant appropriate for the suspected or known pathogen in a predesignated location. The use of sprays is avoided to decrease risk of aerosolizing the pathogen and potentiating spread. Standard operating practices need to be in place to decontaminate the unit.

Once decontaminated, guidelines need to be in place for handling waste that are in compliance with federal regulations, including how medical waste will be packaged, who will transport the waste to the medical waste disposal facility, which medical disposal facilities are used, and the required documentation. Hospitals should create a multidisciplinary team to develop standard protocols for the management of medical waste. This team should include environmental services, infection prevention and control, biosafety officers, hospital administration, and others with expertise in hazardous waste disposal [18].

Intra-facility Transport

Few recommendations and guidelines are published for patient transport within a facility. Once a patient has been admitted to a tertiary facility for care, during the duration of their care, transport outside of the room must be limited as much as possible. Phlebotomy, procedures, and laboratory testing should be limited to the minimum necessary for essential diagnostic evaluation and medical care. Patients may however need further diagnostic testing and management, and while many tests are portable and can be performed at bedside, some diagnostic tests and surgical or invasive clinical interventions will require the patient to be transported to different areas of the hospital. These tests can often be planned ahead, but, in the case of emergent testing or treatment, transport to and from the patient care areas may need to be performed with little notice.

The route to radiology or the interventional suite in the hospital and other locations to which the patient may need to be transported should be predetermined. A mechanism to keep other patients, visitors, and the general public clear of the routes at the time of transport should be established. The path from the room to the testing site needs to be secured by facility staff. This must include identifying an elevator that can be secured to not allow access from other floors until the patient has arrived and the elevator decontaminated [19]. Staff accompanying the patient must be in an appropriate PPE ensemble and knowledgeable of standard operating procedures. The patient can be asked to wear an impervious suit and mask or enveloped in an impervious sheet during transport. The incident response guide at the Bellevue Hospital center has a trained staff walking behind the stretcher and transport team to note possible points of contamination in case a higher level of cleaning or PPE may be required [20]. When necessary, environmental staff should clean the entire transport route including the elevator per hospital cleaning protocols.

If transport or movement outside the isolation room is necessary, the patient should be instructed to wear a surgical mask, if possible, and observe respiratory hygiene. This is a category II recommendation per the CDC guidelines [8]. Category II recommendations are supported by suggestive clinical or epidemiologic studies or a theoretical rationale. For patients with skin lesions associated with varicella or smallpox or draining skin lesions caused by *M. tuberculosis*, the affected areas must be covered to prevent contact or aerosolization of infectious body fluids [8]. This is a CDC category IB recommendation. Category IB recommendations are strongly recommended for implementation and supported by some experimental, clinical, or epidemiologic studies and a strong theoretical rationale. Healthcare personnel transporting patients who are on airborne precautions do not need to wear a mask or respirator during transport if the patient is wearing a mask and infectious skin lesions are covered [8]. Hospital guidelines may differ depending on type of HHCD and its mode of transmission.

Standard operating procedures (SOP) with great attention to detail need to be in place for transport of these at-risk patients within the facility to prevent contamination and spread. PPE and decontamination measures used are dependent on the pathogen involved and mode of spread. Procedures need to be in place for transport of body fluids, blood, and patient care equipment within the facility. Preparations must also be made for unexpected cleanup of spills and body waste during transport.

Ideally patients are kept within their airborne infection isolation room (AIIR), but SOPs should also be in place for emergency evacuation in the case of weather, fire, or other catastrophes. The hospital evacuation plan should be taken into consideration and an evacuation route planned based on minimal exposure to other patients or providers.

Conclusion

While identification and treatment of patients with HHCDs is vital, equally important is the safe transportation while minimizing the risk of spread to the healthcare workers and community. Achieving adequate isolation while transporting from a pre-hospital environment to the healthcare facility and within the facility can be challenging based on mode of spread. Education and training are key for implementation of effective standard- and transmission-based infection control practice in HHCDs. This requires implementation of appropriate administrative policies, work practices, and environmental controls, accompanied by focused education, training, and supervision. Standard operating procedures need to be in place and distributed prior to actual transport to ensure the stakeholders are trained and aware of the policies to ensure a smooth transport with minimal risk.

References

1. Isakov A, Jamison A, Miles W, Ribner B. Safe management of patients with serious communicable diseases: recent experience with Ebola virus. Ann Intern Med. 2014;161:829–30.
2. Centers for Disease Control and Prevention. Hierarchy of controls. Available at https://www.cdc.gov/niosh/topics/hierarchy/. Accessed 1 Mar 2017.
3. Assistant Secretary for Preparedness and Response, Technical Resources, Assistance Center, and Information Exchange. EMS infectious disease playbook. Available at https://asprtracie.hhs.gov/documents/aspr-tracie-transport-playbook-508.pdf. Accessed 30 June 2017.
4. Centers for Disease Control and Prevention. IV. Infection control for prehospital emergency medical services (EMS). Available at http://www.cdc.gov/sars/guidance/i-infection/prehospital.html. Accessed 1 Feb 2017.
5. Isakov A, Miles W, Gibbs S, Lowe J, Jamison A, Swansiger R. Transport and management of patients with confirmed or suspected Ebola virus disease. Ann Emerg Med. 2015;66(3):297–305.

6. Lowe JJ, Jelden KC, Schenarts PJ, Rupp LE, Hawes KJ, Tysor BM, Swansiger RG, Schwedhelm SS, Smith PW, Gibbs SG. Considerations for safe EMS transport of patients infected with Ebola virus. Prehosp Emerg Care. 2015 Apr–Jun;19(2):179–83.
7. Centers for Disease Control and Prevention. Guidance for developing a plan for interfacility transport of persons under investigation or confirmed patients with ebola virus disease in the united states. Available at https://www.cdc.gov/vhf/ebola/healthcare-us/emergency-services/interfacility-transport.html. Accessed 1 Feb 2017.
8. Centers for Disease Control and Prevention. Healthcare Infection Control Practices Advisory Committee (HICPAC). Available at https://www.cdc.gov/infectioncontrol/guidelines/isolation/index.html. Accessed 1 Feb 2017.
9. Occupational Safety and Health Administration. Respiratory protection. Available at https://www.osha.gov/Publications/osha3079.pdf. Accessed 1 Feb 2017.
10. Centers for Disease Control and Prevention. Guidance on personal protective equipment (PPE) to be used by healthcare workers during management of patients with confirmed ebola or persons under investigation (PUIs) for ebola who are clinically unstable of have bleeding, vomiting, or diarrhea in U.S. hospitals, including procedures for donning and doffing PPE. Available at https://www.cdc.gov/vhf/ebola/healthcare-us/ppe/guidance.html. Accessed 1 Feb 2017.
11. Centers for Disease Control and Prevention. Ebola: personal protective equipment (PPE) donning and doffing procedures. Available at https://www.cdc.gov/vhf/ebola/hcp/ppe-training/index.html. Accessed 1 Feb 2017.
12. Occupational Safety and Health Administration. Respiratory protection standard 29 CFR 1910.134. Available at https://www.osha.gov/pls/oshaweb/owadisp.show_document?p_table=STANDARDS&p_id=12716. Accessed 1 Feb 2017.
13. Halpern SD, Emanuel EJ. Ethical guidance on the use of life-sustaining therapies for patients with Ebola in developed countries. Ann Intern Med. 2015;162:304–5.
14. Centers for Disease Control and Prevention. Transport of pediatric patients. Available at https://www.cdc.gov/vhf/ebola/healthcare-us/emergency-services/transporting-pediatric-patients.html. Accessed 1 Feb 2017.
15. American College of Emergency Physicians. Policy statement: medical direction of emergency medical services. Available at http://www.acep.org/Content.aspx?id=29570. Accessed 1 Feb 2017.
16. Assistant Secretary for Preparedness and Response. Planning considerations when developing standard operating procedures for the transfer of an ebola (or other highly infectious disease) patient from/to an air transport provider to/from a ground transport provider. Available at https://www.phe.gov/Preparedness/responders/ebola/Pages/air-transport-factsheet.aspx. Accessed 1 Feb 2017.
17. Fischer WA II, Hynes NA, Perl TM. Protecting health care workers from Ebola: personal protective equipment is critical but is not enough. Ann Intern Med. 2014 Nov 18;161(10):753–4.
18. Hewlett AL, Varkey JB, Smith PW, Ribner BS. Ebola virus disease: preparedness and infection control lessons learned from two biocontainment units. Curr Opin Infect Dis. 2015 Aug;28(4):343–8.
19. Schultz CH, Koenig KL, Alassaf W. Preparing an Academic Medical Center to Manage Patients Infected With Ebola: Experiences of a University Hospital. Disaster Med Public Health Prep. 2015 Oct;9(5):558–67.
20. National Ebola Education and Training Center. Bellevue hospital center incident response guide. Available at https://netec.org/wp-content/uploads/2017/03/Bellevue-EVD-IRG.pdf. Accessed 1 June 2017.

Special Populations: Labor and Delivery 9

John P. Horton

Introduction

Planning for the care of the pregnant patient and fetus is an important facet of clinical care. This chapter will provide a framework to clinical, social, and ethical topics that every facility should consider prior to caring for pregnant patients infected with highly hazardous communicable diseases (HHCD). Pregnancy and fetal care teams include labor and postpartum health nursing, neonatal nursing, obstetricians, pediatricians, anesthesiologists, and the specialists of maternal fetal medicine and neonatology. All must be included and a part of the planning process as each will have a role and specific needs within the care and physical space of consideration. Pregnancy care begins with understanding that there is both a pregnant patient and a fetus. Additionally, one must consider that pregnancy care creates undue fear resulting from lack of knowledge surrounding pregnancy. This fear combined with a desire to avoid harm has the potential to result in lack of appropriate care. At every stage it is important to involve the patient and to address during planning any worries, questions, or fears as it will help to frame the ethical concerns to be answered.

Background

Research, publications, and technical considerations regarding pregnancy care in the setting of HHCDs are sparse. Most case study reports are in field hospitals or low resource environments. While studies in these environments provide valuable lessons, strategies should be reconsidered to include all available resources at each facility. Additionally, pregnant patients may be subject to discrimination leading to

J. P. Horton (✉)
Department of Gynecology and Obstetrics, Division of General Obstetrics and Gynecology, Emory University Healthcare, Atlanta, GA, USA
e-mail: jphorto@emory.edu

A. Hewlett, A. R. K. Murthy (eds.), *Bioemergency Planning*,
https://doi.org/10.1007/978-3-319-77032-1_9

further knowledge gaps. Because of these gaps, any given plan may need to change as information about a particular disease and pregnancy care develops.

Pregnancy may innately change the presentation of a disease or how it can be spread as the chorioamniotic barrier (placenta and membranes) may either create a protected space for amniotic fluid and fetus or possibly serve as a reservoir for infection. Presentation may also be dramatically altered if a disease affects miscarriage rates, placental abruption, rupture of membranes, or precipitation of labor as these conditions may cause significant bleeding, fluid release, and often pain that may not be common for a particular disease. One should never underestimate the amount of bleeding possible at delivery as approximately 750 ml of blood passes through the term pregnant uterus every minute. Control mechanisms for fluid containment need to accommodate for the fact that blood, urine, feces, and amniotic fluid are a part of every delivery as well as the fetal and placental tissues. Caring for a neonate will require plans for not only its protection from disease but also as the neonate may itself serve as a source of contamination.

Facility

The labor and delivery unit should be considered as both a point of access and a possible treatment center. Many women's health units act as mini-hospitals with medical/surgical rooms, intensive care units, surgical suites with preoperative and recovery units, as well as triage and emergent care areas. Labor and delivery units in high resource centers may have an advantage as there are often strict security and monitoring protocols designed to protect newborn access. However, a labor unit has many access points including:

- Direct patient access and reception
- Emergency department
- Direct emergency medical services access
- Nursery/neonatal intensive care unit flow in and out
- Postpartum care flow in and out
- General hospital access points

Screening and sequestration planning should include the above and consideration of the support staff that supply these units with resources. Emergency medical transport teams often bypass emergency department screening measures and may pass through halls and elevators and pass multitudes of patients and staff en route to labor assessment areas.

There are advantages to focusing patient assessment locations to areas that fall outside normal practice patterns. For example, a well-located secure emergency department room may be appropriate for assessment of a laboring patient despite usual practice patterns.

For long-term patient or fetal monitoring, treatment of miscarriage, or labor, a clinical space will need to accommodate multiple people and equipment. When assessing biocontainment units for obstetric needs, one must consider standards for both labor unit rooms and operating theaters. For example, procedures often require space for equipment and multiple people on both sides of the patient as well as both the head and foot of the bed. Current intensive care unit room designs often do not consider the space at the foot of the bed which is necessary in caring for a laboring or miscarrying patient. Preparation must be in place for multiple sources of bodily fluids with copious waste and the need for increased supplies such as towels, linens, or disposable bed absorption mats, recognizing that a balance is needed between being well stocked and overfilling the unit's space.

Specialized equipment needs will vary depending on fetal gestational age and viability and whether fetal monitoring is needed. An ultrasound with supplemental vaginal and abdominal probes that are able to assess intrauterine contents should be available. Many basic ultrasound packages have this ability, but often the necessary probes are not included. Further specific equipment should be available but not stored routinely within the room to decrease need for decontamination.

Obstetric Medications Commonly Needed

1. Pitocin
2. Misoprostol
3. Methylergonovine
4. Carboprost
5. Magnesium sulfate
6. Terbutaline

As a general rule, consider keeping any item that enters the room inside the room until any urgent needs have passed and appropriate decontamination procedures can be completed.

Miscarriage

Many diseases, including those that cause sepsis, increase the rate of miscarriage [1]. This can cause both significant pain and vaginal bleeding that can vary with the gestational age of the fetus. Medical and surgical options for the management of miscarriage should be available. There may be a need for uterine evacuation especially in the setting of an incomplete abortion where some but not all tissue has passed out the uterus. Removal of remaining products of conception can decrease bleeding, improve patient outcome, and decrease bodily fluid output as a source of contamination. Medication such as prostaglandins may be utilized to aid in uterine expression of tissue. Disposable handheld manual vacuum devices can prove useful for early first trimester loss or for the removal of small quantities of retained products of conception. Dilation and evacuation with electric pump suction may be needed and should be available with associated tubing and suction curettes of varying sizes. Having a variety of curette sizes is important for both electric and handheld devices as it allows efficient removal of tissue with the least harm to the patient.

Antenatal Care

Care of a pregnant patient prior to the age of fetal viability will differ little from the average patient. Considerations include medication selection and validating the safety of radiographic studies. Obstetric teams can be consulted for concerns but most care should proceed without change. As example, acute pain management does not differ from established standards, and all efforts should be made to treat pain as aggressively as in standard patient care. Once the age of fetal viability is reached, there will be further testing needed for routine assessment of fetal well-being. Assessment needs may include fetal heart rate monitoring by handheld Doppler or a combined fetal monitoring system that allows for continuous monitoring of fetal heart and uterine contraction activity which involves placement of elastic belts to secure fetal and uterine monitoring probes.

Obstetric Equipment Considerations

1. Ultrasound
   (a) Abdominal Arc Probe
   (b) Vaginal Probe
2. Fetal Doppler
3. Fetal Monitoring system
   (a) Fetal Doppler Probe
   (b) Uterine Tocometer Probe
4. Manual Vacuum Aspirator
5. Electric Suction Device
   (a) Hoses
   (b) Uterine Suction Curettes
6. Under Buttocks Drape with Collection Bag

Because these monitor probes have to be frequently adjusted and repositioned, taping or securing with clear adhesive films is a poor long-term solution, though it may meet an immediate need. Belts that get soiled and need replacing should be exchanged with care to avoid contamination as there is often bodily fluid beneath the patient, and passing a gowned arm or gloved hand under a patient may result in damage to protective gear.

Ultrasound assessment of the fetus may also be needed to help establish gestational age and fetal well-being and to assess for anomalies of fetal anatomy, amniotic fluid levels, and placentation. The ultrasound only needs standard fetal assessment packages though specific probes, such as arc or vaginal types, may be helpful. If available, a single provider that can perform both the patient's physical exam and ultrasound may be beneficial to decrease overall contacts. Radiographic imaging should be limited to those tests that would change medical management to decrease radiation exposure of the fetus and decrease contact exposure. If MRI is desired for further evaluation, the radiologist needs to be aware of pregnancy to take precautions for pregnancy safely. CT IV contrast can be used but MRI IV (gadolinium) contrast should be avoided.

General Labor Considerations

An institution's labor and delivery protocols for care of a pregnant patient with or under investigation for a highly hazardous communicable disease should be discussed and clarified long before the first patient arrives. Technical considerations should begin with assessment of adequate space where a delivery can safely occur to optimize patient care, patient satisfaction, and infection control. Delivery can safely occur without IV access; however, IV access is important for the possible fluid resuscitation and transfusion that may be necessary. Infection alone can increase the rate of postpartum hemorrhage increasing the likelihood of IV fluid needs.

Labor monitoring consists of assessment of cervical dilation as well as fetal heart rate and uterine contractility. The pathogen in question will present different challenges to monitoring. The rate of fetal and amniotic fluid infection may not be known and should be considered as a possible source of contamination. Some pathogens do not routinely cross the chorioamnion barrier, and techniques to decrease vertical transmission to the fetus should be taken. As an example, recommendations for management of women who are infected with hepatitis C include avoidance of artificial rupturing of membranes and avoidance of invasive fetal heat rate monitors as they can increase the likelihood of transmission to the fetus [2]. Assessment of cervical dilation will create a highly soiled glove and sleeve. Extended length gloves such as those used in veterinary medicine can be considered, but commonly found surgical equipment may be more readably available and utilized (Fig. 9.1). Protocols for donning and doffing PPE for vaginal and cervical examination have not been well studied, but protocols decided upon by an institution should be practiced.

Delivery will also present challenges to infection control due to the large quantities of bodily fluid (blood, maternal and fetal urine, and fecal material) present. When choosing PPE, consideration should be given to the significant possibility of bodily fluid projection. As a fetus is delivered, amniotic fluid pressurized by maternal pushing and uterine contraction can jet out of the vagina and travel several feet, including an upward direction. Head and eye protection is an absolute requirement, and impervious headgear may be used to prevent leakage through filters. Umbilical cord clamping and separation should be performed with care and possibly by a birthing assistant to control the loss of blood or potential spray from incising the umbilical cord. Umbilical cord segments to be incised should be devoid of blood as much as possible to avoid blood spray.

Vaginal/Cervical Exam Don Protocol: Over Full coverage PPE

1. Remove outer glove
2. Sanitize
3. Place surgical sleeve over protective outerwear sleeve
4. Sanitize
5. Replace outer glove insuring glove over the sleeve cuff- At all times one should have clear visualization of the outer glove cuff edge, and a buddy system used to monitor.

Vaginal/Cervical Exam Doff Protocol: Over Full coverage PPE

1. Wipe off heavy soil
2. Remove Sleeve From Shoulder pulling downward
3. Sanitize
4. Remove Outer Glove
5. Sanitize. Replace outer glove

At all times one should have clear visualization of the outer glove cuff edge, and a buddy system used to monitor.

Fig. 9.1 Cervical exam PPE protocol proposed at Emory Healthcare

Repairs of minor birth trauma should be weighed with each incidence and assessment of active bleeding, patient sequela, and provider risk. Consideration should be given to the general avoidance of sharps in the case of fluid-borne pathogens. Large lacerations or those that are actively bleeding and in need of repair should only be repaired by experienced providers with judicious use of needles.

Anesthesia

Consultation with anesthesiology is necessary for invaluable insight into pain management. Pain control may be an immediate need with a laboring patient and anesthesiology will provide vital team input. The patient is an important part of the labor team and pain control may assist their ability to maintain cooperation in order to provide a safe delivery environment and decrease infection risks. Common practice for pain control in labor includes IV medication given intermittently or via patient controlled devices and epidural catheter or intrathecal delivered medication. Because these common forms all require needles to gain access and to administer the medication, there is inherent risk to both the patient and practitioner. Depending on the pathogen, there is also a potential risk of introducing infection to a previously uninfected area, such as cerebrospinal fluid (CSF) via epidural or spinal anesthetic techniques.

As a part of preparation, one should assess individual pathogens or conditions that include both blood borne and CSF to plan for the risk involved to the patient and practitioner. The physical space of biocontainment units may also play a role, as full airway management systems may not fit into the allotted space, and IV sedation with mask or manual bag respirator may be required for needed procedures. Anesthesia management systems provide a control that may increase safety for the patient and provider as there is efficient monitoring, delivery of anesthesia, and less physical interaction. It is important to consider the available machines and exactly how a machine would fit through existing passages, be maneuvered into place, and operated safely. Knowing the opportunities and limitations of anesthesia will play a large part in deciding what procedures are possible within a biocontainment space.

Obstetric Emergencies

There are emergencies typical and practiced within the care of pregnancy. Knowing the most common emergencies will allow planning in the setting of highly hazardous communicable diseases. Some clinical pathways to consider include:

- Precipitous delivery
- Postpartum hemorrhage
- Eclampsia seizure
- Fetal heart rate deceleration

Severe postpartum hemorrhage is possible in any delivery and occurs in as many as 4 of 1000 deliveries [3]. Infection increases the likelihood of uterine atony and hemorrhage. Though coagulation disorders can increase the likelihood of bleeding, the bulk of bleeding occurs because the muscle of the uterus has not contracted down after birth. This contractile activity helps to decrease blood flow through arterioles that pass through the uterine wall. Bleeding can be profuse especially in a term pregnancy. The first steps in improving uterine atony include a sweep of intrauterine space to assess for retained tissue and uterine massage to improve muscle tone. One should exercise caution in fluid-borne pathogens as a gloved hand can be passed beyond the glove cuff edge, increasing likelihood of PPE failure. Interventions that should be available to assist include oxytocin, methylergonovine, and carboprost (PGF2 alpha analog); these agents are all in an injectable form and can be administered via IV or IM. Prostaglandins such as misoprostol (PGE1) are helpful as they do not require injection and thusly decrease the need for needles; however, there is a slower onset of action. A kit of the above medications should be present in the biocontainment unit room of a pregnant patient in case hemorrhage occurs. Disseminated intravascular coagulation (DIC) can occur with massive uterine bleeding and should always be considered in postpartum hemorrhage.

Eclampsia is a condition defined by new onset grand mal seizures in a pregnant or postpartum patient that often occur in the setting of preeclampsia but not necessarily with hypertension. The pathophysiology of this condition is complex, but the treatment options for proper preparation and risks of seizure in the setting of communicable pathogens should be discussed. During seizure activity, efforts should be made to maintain the patient safely on the bed and not to restrict movement with physical restraints. Seizures are self-limiting, and the condition is treated with magnesium sulfate via injection IV or IM. A supply of magnesium sulfate should be a part of the obstetric kit.

The treatment of fetal heart rate decelerations includes stopping the administration of uterine stimulants, fluid resuscitation with IV fluid bolus, repositioning of the patient, oxygen administration via nonrebreather mask, and administration of uterine relaxant agents such as terbutaline. If using full-coverage protective garments, care should be taken when repositioning patients to avoid damage or tears of the garment. If fetal heart rate decelerations cannot be corrected, immediate delivery should be considered.

Ethics

No infectious disease plan is complete without consideration of prevention. Women should be counseled on risks that affect their reproductive health and pregnancy outcomes and given opportunity for contraception and disease prevention long before pregnancy occurs. Recent events with regard to H1N1 influenza, Ebola, and Zika highlight the need for extensive and far-reaching education, prevention, and planning for women and men to better understand disease effects upon reproduction. If pregnancy does occur in the setting of a highly hazardous communicable disease, all opportunity should be made to discuss effects on both mother and fetus. Termination should be considered and offered as an option per patient choice. Though ethics committees can be helpful to clarify concerns, nothing replaces patient discussion and the importance of autonomy.

Labor health and pediatric providers are trained extensively to weigh fetal and maternal risks with consideration of delivery. Fetal viability is a convergence where delivery from maternal system and neonatal survival outside the uterus meets. This can be debated intensely and occurs approximately between 22 and 24 weeks in the setting of high resource neonatal intensive care units. Development each day toward 39 weeks gestation may improve neonatal outcome. Institutional ethics councils will be useful to address difficult scenarios when fetal and maternal risks come in conflict with each other. There are diseases for which delivery improves maternal outcome and may spawn plans of premature delivery to optimize maternal outcome. Neonatal outcomes can sometimes be optimized prior to birth and even improved by early delivery. However, neonatal outcomes may be so poor and maternal risk of surgical delivery so high that emergent delivery may not be advisable even in the setting of impending fetal death. Provider safety needs to be considered in the setting of management of a patient with a highly hazardous communicable disease due to the significant chance of contamination. When choices are made that are outside common practice, all team members should be heard and opinions taken with gravity. It is important to also include the patient and their wishes in all medical decision-making and clinical pathways.

Conclusion

Each institution should carefully create its own plan that tailors needs to the facility, equipment, and personnel available. As new facts emerge regarding care and outcomes of pregnant patients with highly hazardous communicable diseases, pathways should be modified as necessary. When creating an obstetric protocol with consideration of biologic contamination, one must go through each step, each movement, each object touched, each piece of equipment utilized, each treatment, and each decision and, most importantly, include as many people as possible to best understand the whole spectrum of care and possible risks.

References

1. Committee on Practice Bulletins-Obstetrics. Practice bulletin no. 183: postpartum hemorrhage. Obstet Gynecol. 2017;130(4):e168–86.
2. Dunkelberg J, Berkley E, Thiel K, Leslie K. Hepatitis B and C in pregnancy: a review and recommendations for care. J Perinatol Off J Calif Perinat Assoc. 2014 Dec;34(12):882–91.
3. Kramer MS, Berg C, Abenhaim H, Dahhou M, Rouleau J, Mehrabadi A, et al. Incidence, risk factors, and temporal trends in severe postpartum hemorrhage. Am J Obstet Gynecol. 2013;209(5):449.e1–7.

Biocontainment Principles for Pediatric Patients

10

Amy S. Arrington

Introduction

Preparing for highly hazardous communicable diseases (HHCD) in healthcare centers must include pediatric hospitals. While much of this preparation is similar between adult and pediatric populations, there are clear differences which must be appreciated when considering the clinical care of the highly infectious pediatric patient, as well as for providing safe and compassionate care for the patient and their families. Specialized biocontainment units, largely funded by academic institutions, have been created to care for children with suspected (person under investigation or "PUI") or confirmed patients with highly hazardous communicable diseases. Care of patients with some pathogens, notably Ebola and other viral hemorrhagic fevers, require the use of special isolation and personal protective equipment by highly trained volunteers representing the interdisciplinary healthcare team including nurses, physicians, respiratory therapists, environmental services, laboratory technologists, and waste management. This was exemplified by the remarkable care of adult patients with Ebola Virus Disease (EVD) in the biocontainment units at the University of Nebraska, Emory, the National Institutes of Health, and Bellevue Hospital. Units that are now capable of caring for children with highly hazardous pathogens, including but not limited to Ebola virus, fully acknowledge their debt to the units that care for adults, but there are notable differences. Developmental issues, parental presence, specialized supplies, and equipment are important considerations when caring for children with suspected or proven EIDs. Currently, there are nine pediatric-specific institutions designated by the CDC as Ebola treatment

A. S. Arrington (✉)
Pediatric Special Isolation Unit, Pediatric Critical Care Medicine,
Texas Children's Hospital, Baylor College of Medicine, Houston, TX, USA
e-mail: amy.arrington@bcm.edu

A. Hewlett, A. R. K. Murthy (eds.), *Bioemergency Planning*,
https://doi.org/10.1007/978-3-319-77032-1_10

Centers, but *all* institutions caring for children should be capable of mastering the tenets of infection prevention and control, biocontainment and isolation of children with a suspected or confirmed HHCD.

Pediatric Specific CDC Designated Ebola Treatment Centers in the United States

- Children's Hospital Colorado; Aurora, Colorado
- Ann & Robert H. Lurie Children's Hospital of Chicago; Chicago, Illinois
- Boston Children's Hospital; Boston, Massachusetts
- Children's Hospitals and Clinics of Minnesota – Saint Paul campus; St. Paul, Minnesota
- Children's Hospital of Philadelphia; Philadelphia, Pennsylvania
- Texas Children's Hospital; Houston, Texas
- Children's Hospital of Wisconsin, Milwaukee; Milwaukee, Wisconsin
- Children's National Medical Center; Washington, D.C.
- Seattle Children's Hospital; Seattle, Washington

Highly Hazardous Pathogens in the Pediatric Population

There are differences between adult and pediatric epidemiology when it comes to highly hazardous pathogens. Here we will briefly examine three of the most recent threatening of the emerging pathogens: SARS-CoV, MERS-CoV, and Ebola virus.

Coronarviruses: Severe Acute Respiratory Syndrome Coronavirus (SARS-CoV) and Middle Eastern Respiratory Syndrome Coronavirus (MERS-Cov)

SARS-CoV

The SARS-CoV epidemic of 2003 is a prime example of how quickly an emerging infectious disease can spread. When reviewing pediatric data available from this epidemic, which occurred from November 2002 through July 2003, the factors most strongly associated with pediatric infections included close contact with adult SARS-CoV patients [1]. In a study looking at pediatric SARS-CoV patients in Toronto, Canada between February and June 2003, SARS-CoV was found to be a relatively mild illness in previously healthy children, resulting in only mild respiratory symptoms, supported in other published reports from pediatric patients from Hong Kong [1–3]. While there were serious diagnostic limitations to these studies, including the lack of serologic data and true confirmation of positive cases, data from all available pediatric studies suggest the majority of pediatric cases had contact with infected adults, resulting in less severe clinical courses in younger patients

(<12 years of age) as compared to teenagers and adult patients, many of whom required mechanical ventilation. SARS-CoV case fatality rate in pediatric patients was estimated to be <1% in patients less than 25 years of age, compared to a case fatality rate of >50% in patients >65 years of age [4].

MERS-CoV

MERS-CoV is a more recently described coronavirus, and while similar to SARS-CoV, presents with more severe clinical symptoms [5]. First isolated in the Kingdom of Saudi Arabia in 2012 from a Saudi businessman who died of pneumonia [6], this respiratory disease has remained primarily isolated to the Arabian Peninsula, with the exception of one significant outbreak in South Korea in 2015 [7]. Isolated from infected camels with confirmed camel-to-human transmission, the exact mode of transmission remains undetermined. Similar to SARS-CoV, hospital acquired infections play an important role in the spread of the virus [5, 8]. Interestingly, a large MERS-CoV outbreak occurred in South Korea in 2015 resulting from the exposure to a *single* infected patient in a crowded emergency room, resulting in MERS-CoV infections in 82 individuals (33 patients, 8 healthcare staff, and 41 visitors), highlighting the need for improved preparedness in early identification and isolation of patients with highly hazardous communicable diseases [8]. Much like with SARS-CoV, pediatric data are limited, as MERS-CoV is primarily a disease seen in the adult population. Of reported pediatric cases, MERS-CoV infections in previously healthy children typically result in non-specific clinical symptoms including fever, cough, shortness of breath and breathing difficulties, and pneumonia, which can progress to acute respiratory distress syndrome and subsequent multi-organ failure [9–12]. From June 2012 through April 2016, only 31 cases (2 known fatalities) of children with MERS-CoV were reported in the Kingdom of Saudi Arabia, compared to a total of 1561 adult cases of MERS-CoV, with 633 fatalities from June 2012 through February 2017. Of the children with more severe symptoms who progressed to death, both had pre-existing conditions (cystic fibrosis and nephrotic syndrome) [10]. Due to non-specific clinical symptoms of both SARS-CoV and MERS-CoV which are similar to other common respiratory pathogens including influenza and Respiratory Syncytial Virus (RSV), a travel and family history is critical in identifying and isolating these patients rapidly upon arrival to any emergency center or primary care setting for proper diagnosis and treatment [13, 14].

Viral Hemorrhagic Fevers: Ebola Virus

Examples of Viral Hemorrhagic fevers in the pediatric population requiring special isolation include Ebola virus, Marburg virus, and Lassa Fever. There is no better example of a viral hemorrhagic fever outbreak than then 2014–2016 Ebola virus disease (EVD) outbreak, which provided new information on pediatric patients with EVD. Much like SARS-CoV and MERS-CoV described above, pediatric patients represented a minority of all patients presenting with suspected or confirmed

EVD. In contrast, the case fatality rate in these children, especially those under 5 years, was quite high, with mortality rates for neonates reaching 100% [15].

Major risk factors for pediatric infections during the 2014–2016 EVD outbreak in West Africa, such as washing of bodies during ritual burials and direct care of sick relatives, were less likely to occur in children and likely partially accounted the lower overall incidence of infection in children, in addition to likely underreporting, and perhaps a faster progression to death in children [16].

In pediatric EVD cases, there is a wide range of symptoms that occur. After an incubation of 2–21 days, these patients usually develop fever, chills, anorexia, headache, and myalgia. In contrast to adults, children more often present with fever and are less likely to report specific complaints of pain, dyspnea, dysphagia, and hiccups. Although designated as a hemorrhagic fever, significant bleeding or bloody diarrhea is seen in a minority of patients. Gastrointestinal involvement predominates after the initial symptomatology, which may include significant diarrhea, emesis, and abdominal pain. It has been suggested that young children are less likely to be able to report such symptoms, which may distort these differences [17].

Special Issues in Pediatric Populations

When preparing for highly hazardous communicable diseases such as SARS-CoV, MERS-CoV, and viral hemorrhagic fevers in pediatric populations, there are special issues facing children and their families which must be carefully considered and include the following:

- General preparedness in pediatric institutions
- Clinical care considerations
- Building a pediatric response team for patients with HHCDs
- Social and ethical considerations specific to the pediatric population
- Pediatric biocontainment unit considerations

General Preparedness in Pediatric Institutions

The majority of pediatric providers will never work in a biocontainment unit, but all frontline providers caring for children should be prepared to <u>identify and isolate</u> suspected patients, as well as rapidly <u>inform</u> the proper individuals if they are faced with a pediatric patient suspected of having a HHCD. Identification of these children with potential exposure to high-risk pathogens can be extremely challenging, particularly in the height of influenza and respiratory virus seasons, where seemingly every child evaluated has symptoms including cough, fever, and diarrhea. Preparedness efforts are therefore time-consuming, costly, and challenging, but potential solutions exist [18]. Travel screening at all points of entry is critical. High-risk travel screening in busy pediatric institutions is a difficult but an essential part of identifying patients with potential HHCDs and properly isolating those patients to limit the spread of disease. Hospitals and clinics should use appropriate travel screening algorithms, ideally built into the electronic medical record admission process and available at all possible points of entry in pediatric centers, including emergency centers, ambulatory clinics, as well as inpatient settings.

While it becomes increasingly difficult in the era of multiple "electronic flags" in the medical record to add another checkpoint for triage, it is necessary to build within these algorithms links to current travel alerts [19]. Additionally, travel screening is useless if positively identified patients are not properly identified and immediately isolated, followed by timely notification of appropriate personnel.

In each institution, pediatric-specific triage screening questions should be developed with the help of infectious disease experts. Example screening questions include:

- "In the past 3 weeks have you or your child traveled outside the U.S. **or** had close contact with someone who traveled outside the U.S.?"
- "Has your child had fever, rash, diarrhea or new skin lesions?"
- "Has your child had difficulty breathing or cough?"
- "Are there ill family members with these symptoms to whom your child was exposed prior to travel?"

Pediatric patients and their caregiver must be promptly isolated if the answers to these questions are "yes" and evaluated by proper experts to determine if the child is indeed at risk for a HHCD requiring special isolation. Immediate isolation requires masking the patient, as well as recognizing that the accompanying family members may also be infected. These identified patients should preferably be placed in a negative pressure room **with their family member/caregiver** to limit exposure to other patients and staff. One nurse and attending physician should assess the patient, and contact should be limited. Once a patient has been identified, isolated, and assessed, internal and external stakeholders must be promptly informed to facilitate testing and, if needed, transport specimens and/or the patient.

Establishing protocols and relationships with all stakeholders in advance is critical to the successful implementation of this process. Attempting to create plans and partnerships during an event is exceedingly difficult and potentially unsafe. In clinical care planning, regional transport partners, waste management groups, and communications experts are essential for successful response to pediatric patients with HHCDs. Informing the proper individuals can be a complex process if not practiced as an institution prior to an event. Creating and maintaining updated telephone trees, developing protocols to rapidly alert health department contacts, and then performing tabletop exercises and simulations to test this communication infrastructure is invaluable to safe and effective care of a patient with a suspected or confirmed highly hazardous communicable disease.

Clinical Care Considerations

All institutions involved in caring for children with suspected or confirmed HHCDs should be capable of offering intensive care for these patients, including mechanical ventilation, management of severe electrolyte disturbances, cardiac arrhythmias, and potentially dialysis in the event of renal failure and/or fluid overload. This requires advanced planning and well defined, well-practiced protocols to provide this level of care both safely and effectively in the setting of special isolation. Having an established, on-call specialized response team who are trained in PPE, protocols, and management of these patients is ideal. Management of critically ill children can be challenging under normal circumstances in the pediatric ICU, but performing procedures and high-level care in PPE is a set of skills which must be practiced.

Building a Pediatric Response Team for Pediatric Patients with Highly Hazardous Communicable Diseases

Careful consideration should be given to choosing healthcare workers for pediatric special isolation teams. While caring for any critically ill child carries specific challenges, the added burden of doing so under the unique stressors of special isolation can be overwhelming, and special attention should be spent on building guidelines and screening tools to ensure that the right team is chosen to care for these special patients and that the proper support is available for the team. In training specialized care teams to care for these children, each institution must decide whether to do this based on the recruitment of volunteers only or if this training is to be mandatory, particularly for staff working in high-risk areas including the emergency center and pediatric intensive care unit. While critical care skills are ideal in the recruitment of these "special response teams," a varied skill set ranging from acute care nurses to ICU nurses, as well as physicians with varied backgrounds, should be considered. Individuals should be carefully screened for behavioral components key to performing well on such a highly specialized team, including the ability to work well with others, self-control, and the ability to remain calm under pressure. In dealing with critically ill children, a pediatric care providers' first instinct is to sacrifice self for patient, and this *cannot* be the case in a caring for a child with a HHCD. The ability to follow strict orders to ensure team safety is key combined with the ability to troubleshoot and think creatively in situations likely never before faced when caring for children. Additionally, members chosen for these specialized teams should undergo full health screens, including potentially fitness and agility testing, as working in personal protective equipment for prolonged periods in environments of high-stress can be incredibly taxing. Human resources should be involved in creating employee policies including sequestration or home monitoring, furlough, pay and benefits, housing for providers, housing for infected employees, food, childcare, and emotional and spiritual support. These actions and policies provide reassurance, a sense of safety, and reduce employee stress. Health and wellness programs and employee assistance programs offering counseling and employee heath teams should be incorporated in the support staff available for all team members of a special response team. Caring for children admitted with HHCDs, potentially in pandemic situations, is likely to cause great amounts of stress, and being able to combat stress and teach caregivers how to manage it is of highest priority in maintaining a healthy team [20].

Social and Ethical Considerations Specific to the Pediatric Population

The social and ethical considerations are complex when dealing with pediatric patients in special isolation, and answers to how these issues should be handled may vary from institution to institution. It is crucial to include the need and stressors of families of these patients, as well as the need to have a plan in place to screen family members for symptoms to both reduce the risk of spread of disease as well as address the needs of adult family members. It must be presumed that if a child is infected with a HHCD, family members are at high risk for exposure and require screening, evaluation, and potentially specialized treatment at an adult treatment center.

The needs of parents and family members of isolated pediatric patients require advance planning, and each institution must decide upon their own policies and procedures prior to facing this situation in real time. First, institutions must decide upon a family visitation policy. These policies can range from several options: first, a "zero tolerance" visitation policy, where families are not allowed inside biocontainment areas but are still provided with video conferencing capabilities in order to interact with their children. Second, family members may primarily spend

time in a separate, designated family room, with only brief visitation to pediatric patients diagnosed with HHCDs. Third, the family or caregiver must remain at the patient's bedside for the entirety of the admission, after demonstrating proper technique in both donning and doffing PPE [21].

As an example, at Texas Children's Hospital in Houston, Texas, a child with a HHCD admitted to the Special Isolation Unit is strictly isolated to prevent further spread of the disease. It is the policy at this institution that parents and family will not be allowed into the unit but are provided with a private family room for respite, where videoconferencing is available. These decisions should be made in consultation with a team including infectious disease experts, state and/or local public health authorities, risk management, and the clinical care staff who will be involved in caring for the child. Additionally, if the decision is made to allow family visitation, this should be closely observed. The ability of families to follow instructions, including appropriate donning and doffing of personal protective equipment, should be carefully considered and may require a case-by-case evaluation. The impact of family visitation must also be balanced with the risk this may bring to staff members caring for the patient. While it is difficult enough to care for a child with a HHCD in full personal protective equipment (PPE), adding family members to the room increases the responsibility of staff to care for and monitor not only the patient, but the family member in addition. It is also important to note that competency in PPE takes practice and suggested quarterly training, and it may be unrealistic to expect family members to be able to don and doff safely without the risk of contamination. Lastly, the decision to allow families to visit children in strict isolation may differ from pathogen to pathogen. The visitation guidelines which apply to a child diagnosed with Ebola virus may differ from those diagnosed with respiratory viruses, such as MERS-CoV.

Regardless of institutional policies, it is critical to address the obvious stress these issues will have upon family members, and it is important to develop policies and procedures to provide exceptional support to these families who are separated from their children, some of whom may be critically ill. This includes specialized training within the care team on ways to care for the family, including assigning "family liaisons," who will serve as a point of contact for the parents and with whom they can develop a trusting relationship regarding the care of their child. The individuals chosen for this position should be excellent communicators and clinical leaders on the patient care team. Parents should be given information on how to obtain updates 24 h a day, with a way to easily communicate with the team caring for their child. Establishing a comfortable, secure, and private space where a family can find solace is recommended. Additionally, family members should be screened daily for symptoms and isolated immediately if there are signs or symptoms of disease.

While local health departments should be partners in the screening of family members, it is important to establish institutional protocols regarding how family will be cared for while their children are patients in special isolation. This includes considering how family will be shielded from media and scrutiny from the general public while entering and exiting the hospital, ensuring families are screened on a daily basis for new symptoms requiring evaluation for potential disease, and monitoring family movements within the hospital to ensure families which may in fact be contagious are confined to specific, controlled areas. This is particularly important with respiratory viruses, such as MERS-CoV and SARS-CoV, where symptoms may initially be vague and patients may be contagious before they are identified.

Caring for the Dying Child in Special Isolation

In caring for critically ill pediatric patients under special isolation, clinical judgment will be required to balance the risks and benefits of heroic therapies as well as the utilization of cardiopulmonary resuscitation (CPR) in the event of cardiopulmonary arrest. This should be decided on a case-by-case basis, always balancing the safety of the care team with the risks of contamination. In pediatrics specifically, children often have little reserve when experiencing severe electrolyte derangements, hypoxemia, and respiratory failure. In many cases, it will be reasonable to offer CPR to patients with these reversible abnormalities [22–24].

Alternatively, if the decision to provide CPR to a child with Ebola virus disease in the setting of massive pulmonary hemorrhage, for example, puts the care team at risk of contamination and infection, the decision to provide CPR should be questioned. These decisions in children are not easy and should be guided by leadership with careful consideration given to the medical team and the psychological effects this discussion will inevitably bring.

In cases of medical futility or the dying pediatric patient in special isolation, offering quality palliative care is not only feasible, but should be discussed prior to the event. Even in the cases where parents and family would not be allowed to visit their dying child (i.e., EVD patients), there are creative ways to involve the family in their child's care. This includes first and foremost offering support, including social work, child life, and chaplain services. Creating "memory tokens" may be useful, though careful consideration must be paid to which items these could be, as only materials which can be successfully autoclaved can be removed from the biocontainment area in cases such as viral hemorrhagic fevers [21]. Photographs and video may assist in helping the family say goodbye, as well as providing items of comfort (e.g., a favorite toy). In the case of some pathogens, such as Ebola virus, it may not be feasible to return these items, and this should be discussed with the family in advance. As with all pediatric end-of-life care, honest and open communication is essential to this process along with allowing the family to grieve, even if isolated from their child. Lastly, the psychological and emotional stress placed on the staff caring for these children must be acknowledged, and staff should be cared for with supportive leadership.

Pediatric Biocontainment Unit Considerations

All institutions caring for pediatric patients should be prepared to either care for a patient who may present after exposure to a highly hazardous pathogen, with basic training in PPE, infection prevention and control and protocols to isolate and care for patients, or have in place protocols to transfer identified patients to facilities where this is care is possible. In this day and age with the ever-expanding ease of international travel, it is crucial to prepare for these patients in advance, including what physical space is necessary to properly isolate and care for these children. In considering the requirements for proper biocontainment of patients with HHCDs, the same principles apply in pediatrics as described previously in the literature [25–28]; however, pediatric-friendly adjustments may need to be made when designing biocontainment units with consideration for pediatric patients.

An example of this is the 8-bed Pediatric Special Isolation Unit built at Texas Children's Hospital. Completed in 2015, this pediatric biocontainment unit exists within a tertiary pediatric hospital and includes all the features of a true biocontainment unit, while remaining pediatric-friendly. Examples of this include a unidirectional workflow in the unit from "clean" to "dirty," specialized air handling systems with negative airflow and HEPA filtration, cleanable surfaces with no grout, pass-through boxes into patient rooms to limit the need for staff entry, a BSL3 laboratory

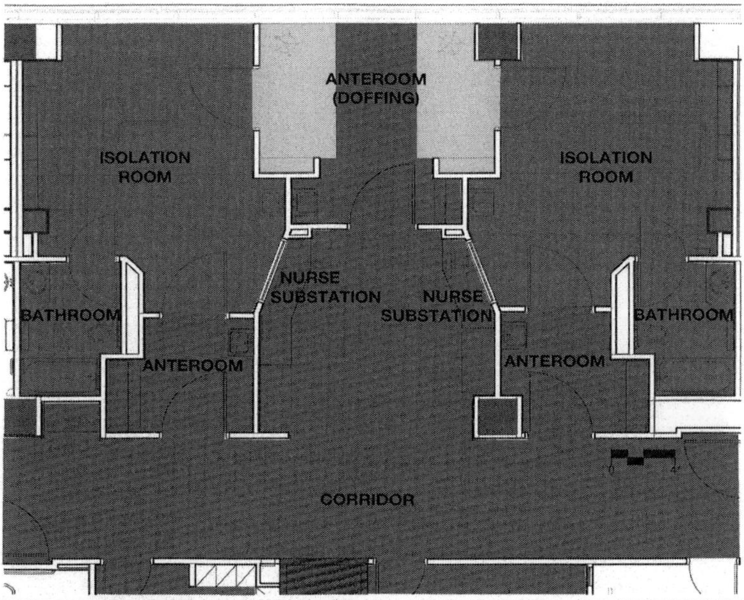

Fig. 10.1 Typical pair of special isolation rooms at Texas Children's Hospital, showing clean (green) to dirty (red) workflow

located within the unit, and three separate pass-through autoclaves capable of processing biohazardous category A waste (Fig. 10.1). Also important in the design of the unit was the ability for parents and families to be able to communicate with their children; therefore cameras were installed to allow family members to observe the room from a dedicated family room, located outside of the unit, when staff feels it is appropriate to do so. Additionally, rooms were built with high visibility so that medical staff could observe both the patient and the staff caring for the child easily from the outside. Rooms were designed in the same bright colors and pediatric themes as typical hospital rooms at Texas Children's Hospital.

Conclusion

Highly hazardous communicable diseases are not a new threat, and as history has shown, they will continue to remain a threat to mankind, both adults and children alike. Critical lessons have been learned in the past regarding how healthcare centers respond to public health emergencies and have highlighted the need for improved infection prevention and control, communication, isolation of HHCD patients, and the ability to care for them in specialized units. While it has been shown in past outbreaks of pathogens ranging from Ebola virus to MERS-CoV that children may be less susceptible to these pathogens, critical illness and/or death can still occur. This requires that all healthcare facilities be prepared to identify, isolate, inform, and potentially provide prolonged care for these most vulnerable of patients and their families. The principles of preparedness in all pediatric institutions are achievable, with planning, practice, and dedication.

References

1. Bitnun A, Read S, Tellier R, Petric M, Richardson SE. Severe acute respiratory syndrome-associated coronavirus infection in Toronto children: a second look. Pediatrics. 2009;123(1):97–101.
2. Li AM, Chan CH, Chan DF. Long-term sequelae of SARS in children. Paediatr Respir Rev. 2004;5(4):296–9.
3. Stockman LJ, Massoudi MS, Helfand R, Erdman D, Siwek AM, Anderson LJ, Parashar UD. Severe acute respiratory syndrome in children. Pediatr Infect Dis J. 2007;26(1):68–74.
4. World Health Organization. Emergency preparedness, response: update 49 – SARS case fatality ratio, incubation period. 2003. http://www.who.int/csr/sarsarchive/2003_05_07a/en/. Accessed 9 Jan 2018.
5. Gao H, Yao H, Yang S, Li L. From SARS to MERS: evidence and speculation. Front Med. 2016;10(4):377–82.
6. Zaki AM, Van Boheemen S, Bestebroer TM, Osterhaus AD, Fouchier RA. Isolation of a novel coronavirus from a man with pneumonia in Saudi Arabia. N Engl J Med. 2012;367:1814–20.
7. Cowling B, Park M, Fang V, Wu P, Leung G, Wu J. Preliminary epidemiological assessment of MERS-CoV outbreak in South Korea, May to June 2015. Euro Surveill. 2015;20:7–13.
8. Cho SY, Kang JM, Ha YE, et al. MERS-CoV outbreak following a single patient exposure in an emergency room in South Korea: an epidemiological outbreak study. Lancet. 2016;388(10048):994–1001.
9. Aleanizy FS, Mohmed N, Alqahtani FY, El Hadi Mohamed RA. Outbreak of Middle East respiratory syndrome coronavirus in Saudi Arabia: a retrospective study. BMC Infect Dis. 2017;17(1):23.
10. Al-Tawfiq JA, Kattan RF, Memish ZA. Middle East respiratory syndrome coronavirus disease is rare in children: an update from Saudi Arabia. World J Clin Pediatr. 2016;5(4):391–6.
11. Thabet F, Chehab M, Bafaqih H, Al Mohaimeed S. Middle East respiratory syndrome coronavirus in children. Saudi Med J. 2015;36:484–6.
12. Memish ZA, Al-Taw q JA, Assiri A, AlRabiah FA, Al Hajjar S, Albarrak A, et al. Middle East respiratory syndrome coronavirus disease in children. Pediatr Infect Dis J. 2014;33:904–6.
13. Shapiro M, London B, Nigri D, Shoss A, Zilber E, Fogel I. Middle East respiratory syndrome coronavirus: review of the current situation in the world. Disaster Mil Med. 2016;2:9.
14. The WHO MERS-CoV Research Group -. State of knowledge and data gaps of Middle East respiratory syndrome coronavirus (MERS-CoV) in humans. PLOS Currents Outbreaks. 2013 Nov 12. Edition 1. https://10.1371/currents.outbreaks.0bf719e352e7478f8ad85fa30127ddb8
15. Kourtis AP, Appelgren K, Chevalier MS, McElroy A. Ebola virus disease: focus on children. Pediatr Infect Dis J. 2015;34(8):893–7.
16. Helleringer S, Noymer A, Clark SJ, et al. Did Ebola relatively spare children? Lancet (London, England). 2015;386(10002):1442–3.
17. Eriksson CO, Uyeki TM, Christian MD, et al. Care of the child with Ebola virus disease. Pediatr Crit Care Med. 2015;16(2):97–103.
18. Saiman L, Arrington AS, Bell M. Preparing for emerging infectious diseases. JAMA Pediatr. 2017;171(5):411–2.
19. Centers for Disease Control and Prevention. Travel health notices. https://wwwnc.cdc.gov/travel/notices.

20. Smith MW, Smith PW, Kratochvil CJ, Schwedhelm S. The psychosocial challenges of caring for patients with Ebola virus disease. Health Secur. 2017;15(1):104–9.
21. Davies HD, Byington CL, Committee on Infectious Diseases. Parental presence during treatment of ebola or other highly consequential infection. Pediatrics. 2016;138(3):pii: e20161891.
22. Johnson DW, Sullivan JN, Piquette CA, et al. Lessons learned: critical care management of patients with Ebola in the United States. Crit Care Med. 2015;43(6):1157–64.
23. Halpern SD, Emanuel EJ. Ethical guidance on the use of life-sustaining therapies for patients with Ebola in developed countries. Ann Intern Med. 2015;162(4):304–5.
24. Leligdowicz A, Fischer WA 2nd, Uyeki TM, et al. Ebola virus disease and critical illness. Crit Care. 2016;20(1):217.
25. Garibaldi BT, Chertow DS. High-containment pathogen preparation in the intensive care unit. Infect Dis Clin N Am. 2017;31(3):561–76.
26. Kortepeter MG, Kwon EH, Hewlett AL, Smith PW, Cieslak TJ. Containment care units for managing patients with highly hazardous infectious diseases: a concept whose time has come. J Infect Dis. 2016;214(suppl 3):S137–41. Epub 2016 Sep 19.
27. Garibaldi BT, Kelen GD, Brower RG, et al. The creation of a biocontainment unit at a tertiary care hospital. The Johns Hopkins medicine experience. Ann Am Thorac Soc. 2016;13(5):600–8.
28. Smith PW, Anderson AO, Christopher GW, et al. Designing a biocontainment unit to care for patients with serious communicable diseases: a consensus statement. Biosecur Bioterror. 2006;4(4):351–65.

Care of Ebola-Infected Human Remains

11

Kate Boulter and Angela Vasa

Postmortem Care of Ebola-Infected Human Remains

The processes involved in the postmortem care of a patient who has succumbed to a highly hazardous infectious disease (HHCD) such as Ebola virus disease (EVD) are high-risk procedures due to the apparent ease in which the disease may be transmitted from the deceased host to the postmortem care provider. Healthcare workers (HCW) and individuals who have a reasonable expectation to participate in the postmortem care of EVD patients must have working knowledge of the inherent risks related to the deceased care process. This chapter describes information gained during the 2014–2016 EVD outbreak, current guidance provided by the CDC to care for EVD-infected remains in hospitals, and how to develop procedures that fit the needs of individual institutions and will conclude with a description of the Nebraska Biocontainment Unit experience while performing EVD postmortem care.

Postmortem Transmission and Viability of Ebola Virus

Ebola virus disease (EVD) is a viral illness caused by exposure to Ebola virus, a highly pathogenic member of the family *Filoviridae*. Exposure occurs when non-intact skin or mucous membranes come in contact with the bodily fluids of an infected person. Once infected with EVD, a person is not highly contagious until they display symptoms of the disease, but as the illness progresses, the risk of transmitting the virus to another person increases as the viral load increases [1]. EVD can result in severe illness with human fatality rates as high as 90% [2]. Patients in the late stages of the disease and non-survivors typically have high viral loads, with

K. Boulter (✉) · A. Vasa
The Nebraska Biocontainment Unit, Nebraska Medicine, Omaha, NE, USA
e-mail: KBoulter@nebraskamed.com

A. Hewlett, A. R. K. Murthy (eds.), *Bioemergency Planning*,
https://doi.org/10.1007/978-3-319-77032-1_11

virus capable of surviving in tissue and body fluids long after the host has died [1], making postmortem care and burial practices high-risk procedures [3]. During the 2014–2016 West African Ebola outbreak, there were reports that up to 70% of the EVD cases in Sierra Leone were linked to persons having unprotected contact with corpses [4]. The World Health Organization suggests that 20% of all new infections are the result of exposure during burial practices [5]. This illustrates that postmortem and mortuary care providers are at high risk for exposure leading to infection and also emphasizes the need for safe postmortem practices. A documented case study in Sierra Leone details how a single fatality was linked to 28 individuals being infected with EVD and how the chain of infection was halted by the establishment of safe burial practices [1]. In this case study, 12 individuals who had contact with the body of the patient after he died, as well as an additional 16 people who had physical contact with him in the days immediately preceding death developed EVD. These first-generation infections had physical contact with the body at a time when the viral load was at its highest while providing end of life care and while performing traditional burial practices that involved prolonged contact through washing, clothing, and preparing the body for internment [1]. These individuals became ill and were cared for by other family members, leading to further second and third generation infections with each additional case having the potential to create new chains of transmission as family members returned to their own homes and villages [1]. The spread of infection in this case study was positively impacted with the implementation of safe burial practices that included community engagement and the utilization of trained burial teams who followed specially designed protocols, thus preventing fourth-generation illnesses in this chain [1]. The study highlights the need for stringent infection prevention and control practices while caring for EVD fatalities in all situations as it has been repeatedly demonstrated that EVD can be transmitted after death.

The stability of Ebola virus in macaque primates infected with EVD and euthanized prior to natural death demonstrated that viable virus remained on the skin of the animals for over a week after they were euthanized [3]. Swab samples taken from nasal mucosa and oral cavities showed that the highest titers of viable virus and viral RNA were found up to 10 weeks postmortem in tissue samples [3]. Humans who die from EVD tend to have high viral loads at the time of their death, making the provision of postmortem care a high-risk procedure requiring stringent infection control practices to prevent exposure and further spread of the disease [2].

To assist in controlling the spread of EVD from burial practices in Africa, the World Health Organization developed and published the guide "Field Situation: How to conduct safe and dignified burial of a patient who has died from suspected or confirmed Ebola virus disease" [6]. The guide was developed for burial teams involved in the management of the deceased who were confirmed or suspected to have died from EVD in hospitals, clinics, or in their homes. This manual provides directions on how to respect the traditions and customs of the grieving families and friends while ensuring safe and dignified burials through a written and pictogram 12-step process [6].

Fortunately, the experience encountered within the United States and other developed countries during the EVD outbreak did not include the devastating community effects that West African countries endured. However, healthcare workers who provided care for those patients who were repatriated or traveled to these countries had to be prepared and equipped to handle EVD-infected human remains safely to protect themselves and the communities in which they live. Preparation plans should be made in collaboration with local and state public health and must comply with all associated rules and regulations.

CDC Guidance

In 2014, the Centers for Disease Control and Prevention (CDC) published recommendations for personnel involved in the postmortem care of EVD-infected remains. These guidelines provide a detailed process for postmortem preparation, transportation, and the disposition of human remains. Key points include not washing or cleaning the body, leaving medical equipment and devices in place, not embalming the body, and avoiding autopsy unless absolutely necessary; if an autopsy is deemed necessary, the CDC must be included in the planning process [7]. The CDC published guidelines for postmortem preparation of the body in a hospital room that details the recommended actions for how to place the body within three different standards of cremation-compatible mortuary bags prior to transportation for cremation or internment. The high risk to personal health dictates that this process should only be performed by personnel trained in the handling of EVD-infected human remains [8]. It also requires sectioning the working area into "hot" and "cold" zones. The hot zone (likely the patient room) is the area in which the body will be placed into the mortuary bags. This area is likely to have contaminated surfaces. The cold zone is an adjacent area that is free from contamination secondary to stringent infection control procedures. Considerable care must be taken when performing the transfer process from the hot to the cold zone to avoid cross contamination and involves two separate teams. The first team will prepare and contain the body in the mortuary bags within the designated hot zone, and the second team will receive the contained remains in the cold zone and proceed with transportation to the crematorium or place of burial. The process should be executed in a cautious manner that allows for adequate time to safely complete each step. There is specific equipment, some of which is not normally found in a hospital unit, that is required throughout the packaging process such as heat-sealable chlorine-free material, mortuary bags that meet a minimum criterion, a heat wand, and dedicated scissors (Table 11.1). It is essential and worth emphasizing that prior to performing the procedure, training on both hot and cold zone tasks be provided to all personnel involved in the process. Training should include safe and effective PPE donning and doffing with demonstrated competency in the procedures. It is also advised to have plans in place to address unforeseen events such as a body fluid spill or healthcare worker exposure to body fluids. Once the remains have been secured within the

Table 11.1 Equipment recommended by the CDC for Ebola-infected remains

Item description	Location details	Comments
A hospital gurney	Prepared in the cold zone and transferred into the hot zone.	Prepare the gurney with three cremation-compatible mortuary bags opened and ready to receive the remains. The order to place the mortuary bags on the gurney is in the reverse order in which the body will be placed into them.
First mortuary bag (must be cremation compatible)	Taken into the hot zone on the gurney. The CDC process involves removing this mortuary bag from the gurney to place the linen-wrapped body into it on the bed and then transfer it back to the gurney after it has been closed and disinfected.	The mortuary bag should be made from vinyl or other chlorine-free material with a minimum thickness of 6 mil (152 micrometers). It must have factory-sealed or factory-welded seams to prevent fluid leaks and a zipper closure on top. When securing the zipper, efforts should be taken to prevent creating an air bubble inside the mortuary bag that when pressure is applied to the bag may cause aerosolization of the virus from inside the bag. Handle this mortuary bag with care when transferring it from the bed back to the gurney as lifting it may cause the bag to rip from the weight of the body. The team performing this step should consider the use of a transfer device if available.
Thermal sealer	Hot zone	The thermal sealer must plug into an electrical outlet in the hot zone that will allow the cord to reach the entire circumference of the bed. Determine a safe location for placing the thermal sealer when not in use and ensure all personnel know when it is switched on. Extreme caution must be taken when using the thermal sealer as heat generated by the thermal sealer has potential to burn through PPE if handled incorrectly. Small clamps that may be purchased in any hardware store can assist in the sealing process by holding the edges of the bag to be sealed in a way that hands can avoid being in close proximity to the thermal sealer.
Second mortuary bag (must be cremation compatible)	Taken into the hot zone on the gurney.	The middle and second layer mortuary bag must be made from chlorine-free material that is impervious to fluids and can be heat-sealed using the thermal sealer around the body to form a leak-proof pouch. When sealing this bag, create a double seal so that the outermost seal can be cut through the middle of its entire length to provide a perfectly sealed edge without any open areas. Use caution when handling the cut material as the remaining edge will be sharp, especially on the corners Note: If the material chosen provides instructions on where to make the seals, it is advisable to determine if the markings indicate how the edges should be sealed for the containment of highly hazardous communicable diseases or if they are there for alternate use. If these markings apply to alternate use scenarios, the markings should be disregarded and included in staff training for using the material to adhere to current CDC guidelines.

(continued)

Table 11.1 (continued)

Item description	Location details	Comments
Third mortuary bag (must be cremation compatible) This bag is widely known as a heavy-duty mortuary bag	Taken into the hot zone on the gurney. Once all mortuary bags are sealed and disinfected within this bag, it is closed, disinfected, and transferred to the clean zone.	Must be constructed from laminated vinyl or other chlorine-free material with a minimum thickness of 18 mil (457 micrometers) with factory-heat-sealed or factory-welded seams to prevent leakage. It must have handle straps made from reinforced material that are secured by rivets (not stitched) and be reinforced with handle straps that run under the pouch to support the underside when transferring to prevent the bag ripping from pressure put on the handles during the move. The zipper should be on the top and contain two sliders that allow the bag to be locked with a zip tie.
Scissors	Hot zone	Scissors for cutting through the outermost seal on the second mortuary bag. Consider using trauma shears to prevent having sharp points as a hazard to staff.
Camera or mobile phone capable of securely transferring photographs electronically	Hot zone	Consult with your designated facility compliance office to ensure compliance with federal, state, and your institutional regulations, as facial photographic images of patients are protected health information.

mortuary bags and the external surfaces disinfected, personnel wearing single-use disposable gloves with extended cuffs and a long-sleeved disposable gown can proceed with transportation.

Transporting Ebola-Infected Human Remains

The US Department of Transportation regulates the transportation of infectious substances and categorizes it into two main groups: Category A and Category B infectious substance. Category A infectious substances are defined as: “A material known or reasonably expected to contain a pathogen, such as Ebola, that is in a form capable of causing permanent disability or life threatening or fatal disease in otherwise healthy humans or animals when exposed to it” (HMR) (49 CFR, Parts 171–180) [9].

Any substance meeting this definition is subject to the US Department of Transportation’s Hazardous Materials Regulations (HMR) and must be treated as Category A hazardous waste.

Category B infectious substances are classified as regulated medical waste that do not meet the criteria to be included as Category A and thus do not require the same special handling.

To determine the appropriate category for human remains, the Department of Transportation provides this definition: "An infectious substance classification is based on the patient or animal's known medical history or symptoms, endemic local conditions, or professional judgment concerning the individual circumstances of the source human or animals" [9].

Using this definition it could be assumed that transporting EVD-infected human remains is subject to the US Department of Transportation's HMR and as such would be considered Category A infectious substance. However, as long as the human remains are being transported for cremation, interment, or medical research, they are exempted from HMR 49 CFR, Parts 171–180, [7] and are not subject to Category A transportation regulations. It is recommended, however, that the transport route be determined in advance and in collaboration with all relevant authorities. Consideration should be given to limiting the transition time from the point of containment to the crematorium or place of burial, as well as how the chain of custody will be maintained throughout the transportation. If the transport plan involves interstate movement, it must be coordinated with the CDC Emergency Operations Center (EOC) by calling the designated number found on the CDC website [7].

The CDC recommends having the following available during the transportation:

- A biohazard spill kit with recommended PPE required for cleaning EVD spills
- An EPA-registered hospital disinfectant
- Biohazard waste bags

As a precaution, if a spill were to occur, transportation personnel should be trained in the spill cleanup process and in how the waste generated will be disposed of. Additionally, although the remains are not subject to HMR 49 CFR, the CDC guidance directs that infectious substance labels be applied to the external mortuary bags [7] (Table 11.2).

Table 11.2 Transportation labels

United Nations UN 2814 Infectious Substance Affecting Humans label	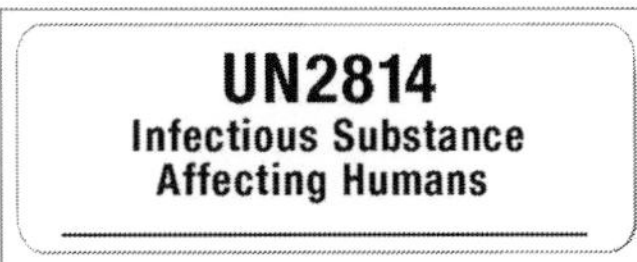
A 'Do Not Open' label	
A label with the name and phone number of the hospital administrator	
US Department of Transportation **Hazmat** 6 Infectious substance	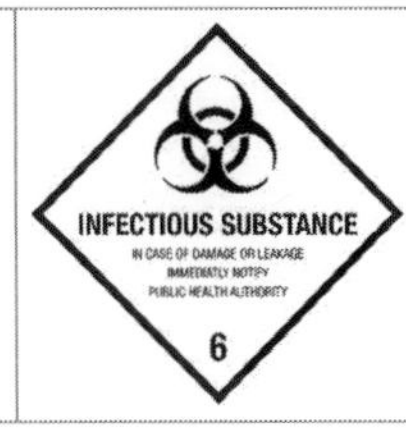

The Disposition of EVD-Infected Human Remains

The CDC advises that EVD remains should be cremated. Once the body has been cremated, the ashes are no longer considered infectious and can be handled in accordance with normal procedures. There are instances however when cremation cannot be performed due to potential hazards such as the presence of implanted electronic medical devices that have the potential to explode in the retort. In such an instance, burial is considered an acceptable alternative. If burial is the chosen method it should be performed using a standard metal casket in accordance with state and local burial regulations. The casket containing the triple bagged remains can be handled without PPE [7].

The Nebraska Biocontainment Unit Process

The Nebraska Biocontainment Unit (NBU) method for containing EVD infected human remains considers the minimum standards recommended by the CDC, but is individualized to fit the physical needs of the NBU. This amended process utilizes the required mortuary bags plus an additional heavy-duty mortuary bag. It also includes modifcations on how to transition the remains from the hot zone, to the warm zone, to the cold zone, and then out of the NBU. Process steps follow strict infection control measures that ensure there is no contamination across work zones (Fig. 11.1). The deliberate use of multiple teams for each zone (hot, warm, cold) and specific tasks for each team reduces the potential for error when transferring the remains out of the patient care area. The Nebraska standard operating procedure (SOP) maintains the delineation of zones by limiting the amount of equipment that is utilized in each zone (Table 11.1). The remains are initially wrapped in bed linens and placed into a standard postmortem bag and then the heat-sealed chlorine-free material following the CDC guidelines on the sealing process. The remains are then passed out of the room to the team in the warm zone using a vertical slide technique at the patient room door into the third protective layer that consists of a heavy-duty mortuary bag (Fig. 11.2). It is critical at this point to ensure that the hospital bed that remains within the hot zone boundary and the gurney that remains in the warm zone do not touch in order to decrease the risk of cross contamination. A slide board is used to bridge the bed to the gurney, and when the remains are slid over, the slide board is pulled into the hot zone where it will await disinfection. The hot zone door is closed, and the team in the warm zone closes the heavy-duty mortuary bag and disinfects it with an EPA-approved disinfectant. The remains are then wheeled to the warm/cold zone transition to a third team, and the vertical slide technique is again utilized and the remains secured into the outermost heavy-duty mortuary bag that is immediately secured and disinfected by the NBU team in the cold zone. These packaged remains are then transferred into the custody of the mortuary service provider who ensures their safe transport for final disposition. To maintain chain of custody, an NBU team member also accompanies the remains to the crematorium.

Mortuary Guidance Job Aid: Postmortem Preparation in a Hospital Room

Appropriate personal protective equipment (PPE) must be worn while performing these tasks.

1. Turn on thermal sealer.
2. Use digital camera or mobile phone to take a photograph of the deceased's face. Send photo via Wi-Fi, e-mail, or text message to site manager through secure means. Decontaminate or properly discard camera or mobile phone.
3. Position gurney with three pre-opened body bags next to hospital bed.
4. Pull bed sheet(s) up and around body. Do not wash or clean body. Do not remove inserted medical equipment from body.
5. Remove first bag from gurney. Gently roll body wrapped in sheets while sliding first bag under body.
6. Complete transfer of body to first bag. Zip up bag. Minimize air in bag.
7. Disinfect gloved hands using alcohol-based hand rub (ABHR). If any areas of PPE have visible contamination, disinfect with an EPA-registered disinfectant wipe.
8. Disinfect outside of first bag with an EPA-registered hospital disinfectant.
9. Transfer first bag with body to gurney, placing it on top of second bag.
10. Disinfect gloved hands using ABHR.
11. Fold second bag around first bag and heat seal approximately 2" from edges. Remove air from second bag. Heat seal bag again approximately 1" below initial seal and heat seal diagonally across corners. Use scissors to trim off any excess material along seam. Turn off or unplug thermal sealer. Decontaminate thermal sealer before it is removed from hot zone or reused.
12. Disinfect outside of second bag with EPA-registered hospital disinfectant.
13. Disinfect gloved hands using ABHR.
14. Work third bag around second bag. Zip up third bag. Zip tie the zipper shut.
15. Disinfect gloved hands using ABHR.
16. Wheel gurney to decontamination area.
17. Decontaminate surface of body bag with EPA-registered hospital disinfectant.
    - Begin by applying the hospital disinfectant to top of bag and any exposed areas of gurney's cot.
    - Roll bag to one side to decontaminate half of bottom of bag and newly exposed portion of gurney's cot.
    - Repeat with other side of bag and gurney.
    - After visible soil has been removed with EPA-registered disinfectant wipe, reapply EPA-registered hospital disinfectant and allow sufficient contact time, as specified by manufacturer.
18. Disinfect surfaces of gurney from handles to wheels with an EPA-registered hospital disinfectant.
19. Disinfect gloved hands using ABHR.
20. Push gurney so only gurney and decontaminated body bag enter cold zone. Do not enter cold zone. A new set of workers will receive the body.
21. Proceed to PPE removal area.

For more information: Guidance for Safe Handling of Human Remains in U.S. Hospitals and Mortuaries. http://www.cdc.gov/vhf/ebola/healthcare-us/hospitals/handling-human-remains.html

DEPARTMENT OF HEALTH AND HUMAN SERVICES
Centers for Disease Control and Prevention
National Institute for Occupational Safety and Health

Fig. 11.1 CDC mortuary guidance job aid (An electronic version can be obtained at https://www.cdc.gov/vhf/ebola/pdf/postmortom-preparation.pdf)

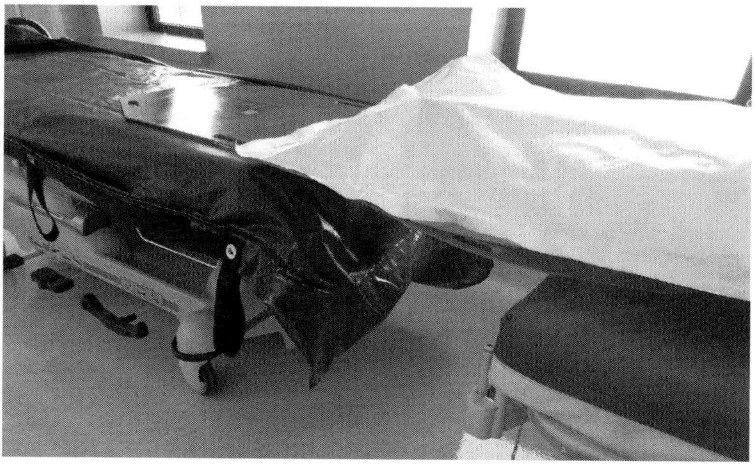

Fig. 11.2 Nebraska Biocontainment Unit vertical slide technique

The process used by the NBU is tailored to accommodate the architecture and engineering controls of the unit. NBU team members receive education on all SOPs as well as the opportunity to practice these techniques during training, exercises and drills. All institutions may have unique situations to which it will require them to adapt the guidelines and develop a process that will meet their needs to provide safe postmortem care of EVD remains.

The Development of Standard Operating Procedures

It is crucial to have standard operating procedures (SOPs) in place to guide healthcare professionals who may be asked to handle the remains of a person who has succumbed to EVD. The incorporation of SOPs contributed to the increased safety of the burial practices used in West Africa. According to a Morbidity and Mortality Report released by the CDC in 2015, findings from a national assessment of burial practices were used to inform the development of a national SOP for safe, dignified medical burials. The national implementation of this SOP might have made dignified burial safer and increased the community support for these practices [10]. When developing SOPs for facility-specific practices, consideration should be given to any policies and procedures that currently exist, as well as the most up-to-date guidance available from expert sources, such as the Centers for Disease Control and Prevention [7] (see Fig. 11.1). The guidelines published by the CDC are meant to serve as a basis from which institutions can build their own individualized protocols. It is imperative to ensure that these procedures include detailed high-level infection control measures that will protect the staff handling the remains, the hospital environment, and the community from any potential contamination from the decedent. The SOPs should provide direction to personnel in the patient care area as well as include references for collaborating partners. SOPs are a great tool to drive the provision of care, but they are only beneficial if personnel know and understand them. The incorporation of exercises and training is an important step in developing a program that includes safe handling of infectious remains.

Training and Exercise

The use of exercises takes preparedness one step further by providing a safe way to practice the plan before an incident occurs, document strengths, and identify areas for improvement within the process [11]. Exercises are a focused practice activity that places participants in a simulated situation, requiring them to function in the capacity that would be expected in a real event [11]. There are many steps to preparing the remains of a person with EVD, and training personnel ahead of time can help to mitigate the stress response that may be experienced during an actual event. When planning an exercise or a drill to test the protocols related to care of the deceased, attention should be paid to providing reality-based scenarios, injects, and outcomes. One important aspect is the use of a human patient simulator that is similar in size and weight to an average person. The steps of the packaging process that include lifting the remains and sliding them into the next layer can be taxing and cause damage to the mortuary bags if not done correctly. Allowing personnel to experience an adverse incident during a controlled drill encourages critical thinking and the opportunity to strengthen the SOP in use.

The handling of the remains of EVD patients is considered a high-risk procedure due to the exceedingly high level of viremia that remains present postmortem. This classification requires healthcare professionals to carefully consider what type of personal protective equipment (PPE) to wear when performing these tasks. When performing any tasks related to handling decedent remains, the CDC recommends the use of PPE that covers all of the provider's skin and mucous membranes. This ensemble includes an impermeable gown or coveralls, respiratory protection including powered air purifying respirator (PAPR) or N95 respirator with a face shield and shoulder length head covering, single-use disposable boot covers, two pairs of single-use extended cuff gloves, and a single-use disposable apron [8]. The decision on what PPE to use in this type of care takes into account the volume of bodily fluids present, the safety and comfort of the staff, and the risk posed by the tasks being performed. The Nebraska Biocontainment Unit opted to use PAPR level PPE when handling the remains of a patient with EVD (Fig. 11.3). The use of PAPR level PPE provided staff with the appropriate level of protection and comfort needed to safely contain the EVD remains. The use of this type of PPE demands that healthcare personnel have advanced training. When planning training for staff to exercise SOPs addressing the handling of infectious remains, the incorporation of the required PPE is a critical element, as the act of donning and doffing PPE is complex and requires strict attention to detail.

In addition to internal departmental collaboration, conversations with local and state public health departments should occur as these SOPs are being drafted and

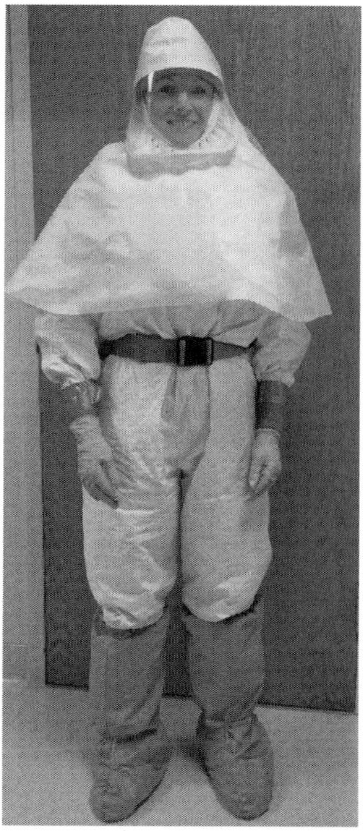

Fig. 11.3 Nebraska Biocontainment Unit, powered air purifying respirator (PAPR) level PPE

exercised. The level of public health involvement can vary greatly by geographical region, so establishing role and responsibility expectations prior to an event will enhance the safety and efficiency of the response. In response to the 2014–2016 EVD outbreak, the newly established Regional Ebola and other Special Pathogen Treatment Centers across the United States developed both state and regional concepts of operations (CONOPS). Included in these CONOPS are provisions for the safe transport and disposition of remains within respective areas. Facilities that are independently crafting SOPs should consider obtaining the most current copy of the applicable CONOPS to ensure a cohesive and robust approach.

Memorandum of Understanding

Another focal point that requires advanced consideration is the creation of contracts or memorandums of understanding (MOUs) with key partners. The US Agency of International Development (USAID) defines an MOU as "a signed non-obligating and legally non-binding document that describes the intentions of the alliance members to work together to address a shared development challenge" [12]. When creating plans to address the handling of infectious remains, it is imperative to consider the final disposition and which community partners are willing or available to assist.

The recommended final disposition of the remains of persons with confirmed EVD is either cremation or the interment of the remains using an approved metal casket [7]. This recommendation drives the suggestion that any facility with a reasonable expectation to provide care for the patients with EVD or other highly hazardous communicable disease initiates steps to form MOUs with local crematoriums, mortuary service providers, and cemeteries. There are many benefits to having MOUs in place in advance of an event to formalize community partnerships. Having an MOU can help to ensure that all participating parties agree on their roles and responsibilities, thus decreasing misunderstandings and potential future conflicts. An MOU also serves as an outline for how the partnership will be utilized during times of need and many times represents the only document that formalizes the relationship between the respective agencies. Since these documents are not legally binding, it is also beneficial to maintain positive working relationships with identified key partners. One of the difficulties noted during the care of patients with EVD in the United States was the reluctance of crematoriums and funeral service providers to commit their services in the midst of the outbreak.

The Nebraska Biocontainment Unit created an MOU with a local crematorium as part of initial protocol development. The existence of this MOU served to expedite and ensure the safe containment, transport, and disposition of patient remains. An important point to consider is the need to protect the identity of community partners if desired. The decision to participate in the disposition of the remains of a decedent due to a highly hazardous communicable disease could potentially impact business revenue due to public perception and fear. Facilities should have an understanding of these expectations and respect the wishes of their community partners. These expectations should be clearly identified in advance when drafting the MOU.

Behavioral Health and Emotional Support

Staff

The loss of a patient in any setting can be emotionally challenging for HCWs. This loss is intensified when the care efforts of an entire unit are solely focused on one patient, as was often the case with EVD patients treated in the United States and other developed countries. When staff were interviewed to discuss the emotional impact of providing care in a biocontainment unit, ten HCWs (50%) identified the death of their patient as the most taxing event of the whole experience [13]. One approach to help support personnel after the death of a patient is acknowledging the pain of the event and providing a safe space to grieve the loss. It is important to obtain input and assistance for the HCWs from a trained behavioral health professional. The facilitation of a private memorial service honoring the person who passed as well as the heroic efforts of the team can provide much needed solace. It is within this shared space of grief that the healing process can begin.

Support for Family and Significant Others

The psychosocial needs of family members and significant others are paramount when providing care after the death of a patient. This is even more profound when the patient in question has fallen victim to a highly hazardous communicable disease. These patients are placed in strict isolation, and contact with their family member is either severely limited or nonexistent outside of a video connection. The inability to touch, hold, or caress a loved one when death is imminent can serve to compound the loss and extend the grieving process.

In the event of a patient's death, establishing the ability to support the needs of the family is imperative. The ability to view the body using telehealth programs can provide necessary closure for the patient's family. If the family has a religious affiliation or preference, consideration should be given to saying prayers together when appropriate or administering a blessing which can be supported using technology. Given that private communication in these instances can be very limited, it may be helpful for staff to include letters written by the family when preparing the remains. This allows for the expression of private thoughts that can stay between the family and the patient. Additionally, if cremation is determined to be the final disposition of the patient, the return of the ashes to the family should be considered. Consideration should also be given to returning the patient's belongings that can be effectively decontaminated to family members.

Conclusion

The postmortem care of Ebola virus-infected human remains is a hazardous procedure and must be performed with a high level of attention to infection control practices utilizing specialized equipment. Healthcare facilities should develop SOPs and MOUs with community partners that take into account their own unique circumstances. Training and exercising the SOPs is essential in order to maintain preparedness and proficiency. It is important to maintain the decedent's dignity at the end of life by taking efforts to treat the deceased patient and his or her family with respect and kindness and to provide behavioral health support for family members as well as HCWs involved in the patient's care.

References

1. Curran KG, Gibson JJ, Marke D, Caulker V, et al. Cluster of Ebola virus disease linked to a single funeral – Moyamba District, Sierra Leone, 2014. Morb Mortal Wkly Rep. 2016;65(8):202–5.
2. Rewar S, Mirdha D. Transmission of Ebola virus disease: an overview. Ann Glob Health. 2014;80(6):444–51.
3. Prescott JB, Bushmaker T, Fischer RJ, Miazgowicz K, Judson SD, Munster VJ. Postmortem Stability of Ebola Virus. Emerg Infect Dis. 2015 May;21(5):856–9.

4. Maxmen A for National Geographic. How the fight against Ebola tested a culture's traditions. Online at http://news.nationalgeographic.com/2015/01/150130-ebola-virus-outbreak-epidemic-sierra-leone-funerals/. January 30, 2015 [Retrieved 4 Feb 2017].
5. World Health Organization. New WHO safe and dignified burial protocol – key to reducing Ebola transmission. Online at: http://www.who.int/mediacentre/news/notes/2014/ebola-burial-protocol/en/. November 7, 2014 [Retrieved 25 Feb 2017].
6. World Health Organization. Field situation: how to conduct safe and dignified burial of a patient who has died from suspected or confirmed Ebola virus disease. Online at: www.who.int/csr/resources/publications/ebola/safe-burial-protocol/en/ October 2014 [Retrieved 11 Mar 2017].
7. CDC. Guidance for safe handling of human remains of Ebola patients in U.S. hospitals and mortuaries. Ebola Virus Disease. Online at: https://www.cdc.gov/vhf/ebola/healthcare-us/hospitals/handling-human-remains.html February 11, 2015 [Retrieved 25 Feb 2017].
8. CDC. Guidance on Personal Protective Equipment (PPE) to be used by healthcare workers during management of patients with confirmed Ebola or Persons under Investigation (PUIs) for Ebola who are clinically unstable or have bleeding, vomiting, or diarrhea in U.S. hospitals, including procedures for Donning and Doffing PPE. Ebola Virus Disease. Online at: https://www.cdc.gov/vhf/ebola/healthcare-us/ppe/guidance.html. November 17, 2015 [Retrieved 10 Mar 2017].
9. U.S. Department of Transportation. Department of transportation guidance for transporting Ebola contaminated items, a category A infectious substance. PHMSA Pipeline and Hazardous Materials Safety Administration. Online at: http://phmsa.dot.gov/hazmat/transporting-infectious-substances/packaging-of-ebola-contaminated-waste/faq October 1, 2012 [Retrieved 4 Mar 2017].
10. Nielsen C, Kidd S, Sillah A, Davis E, Mermin J, Kilmarx P. Improving Burial Practices and Cemetery Management during an Ebola Virus Disease Epidemic — Sierra Leone, 2014. Morb Mortal Wkly Rep (MMWR), January 16 2014. Online at: https://www.cdc.gov/mmwr/preview/mmwrhtml/mm6401a6.htm.
11. Kunes T. The importance of exercises to effective incident response. Kestrel Management. March 12, 2017. Online at: http://kestrelmanagement.com/importance-exercises-effective-incident-response/.
12. United States Agency for International Development. Memorandum of Understanding (MOU). March 11, 2017. Online at: https://www.usaid.gov/sites/default/files/documents/1880/Section%206%20MOU%20Overview.public.updated022013.pdf
13. Smith M, Smith PW, Kratochvil C, Schwedhelm M. The psychosocial challenges of caring for patients with Ebola virus disease. Health Security. 2017;15(1):104–9.

Evaluation of the Person Under Investigation

12

Paul D. Biddinger and Erica S. Shenoy

Introduction and Background

The ability to detect and diagnose patients infected with a highly hazardous communicable disease (HHCD) must be a priority for healthcare facilities in order to limit the morbidity and mortality of infection and to ensure the safety of staff and other patients through the early initiation of appropriate infection prevention measures. A patient presenting to healthcare facilities with specific clinical and epidemiological risk factors for infection with one of these pathogens may be termed a person under investigation (PUI) for the disease, and healthcare staff should utilize carefully developed protocols and procedures to guide their subsequent isolation and clinical evaluation practices until the disease has been ruled in or out.

Unfortunately, many factors challenge the appropriate early identification and appropriate isolation of PUIs in practice. These include lack of familiarity with PUI definitions and lack of knowledge regarding necessary actions once a PUI is suspected or identified. In addition, evolving PUI definitions from public health authorities, as well as changes in clinical guidance regarding recommended actions, as can occur with a new or newly emerging pathogen, further complicate PUI assessment. Inadequate early implementation of appropriate infection prevention measures can have severe consequences, and prior delays have resulted in nosocomial transmission [1–6].

P. D. Biddinger (✉)
Department of Emergency Medicine, Center for Disaster Medicine, Region 1 Ebola and Other Special Pathogens Treatment Center, Massachusetts General Hospital, Boston, MA, USA
e-mail: pbiddinger@partners.org

E. S. Shenoy
Infection Control Unit, Division of Infectious Diseases, Region 1 Ebola and Other Special Pathogens Treatment Center, Massachusetts General Hospital; Harvard Medical School, Boston, MA, USA

A. Hewlett, A. R. K. Murthy (eds.), *Bioemergency Planning*,
https://doi.org/10.1007/978-3-319-77032-1_12

Therefore, rational and thoughtful approaches to identifying, evaluating, and providing care for HHCD PUIs are essential. Healthcare facilities must support vigilance in the suspicion of these diseases and support safe and effective care for all patients. Plans developed to support the evaluation of PUIs must also minimize the potential disruptions to routine facility operations, since PUIs will most likely outnumber actual confirmed cases, creating substantial operational and economic costs for institutions if not managed efficiently. The identify-isolate-inform framework introduced by the CDC during the 2014–2016 Ebola virus disease (EVD) outbreak can serve as a basic framework upon which further planning for the evaluation of PUIs for any HHCD, not just EVD, and can be used in any setting [7]. In this chapter, we will discuss features of PUI definitions and their implementation by healthcare providers, the various clinical settings that may be used for evaluation of the PUI, an approach to PUIs using the identify-isolate-inform framework, the specific evaluation and management methods that may be used in evaluating PUIs, and the clinical and operational challenges encountered during evaluation and management. We will conclude with a look to the ongoing challenges in PUI evaluation and areas where future advances in knowledge and policy are needed.

Understanding and Applying PUI Definitions

Evaluation of the PUI requires an understanding of each of the factors required to meet the definition. For well-known diseases, the term clinically compatible case [8] may sometimes be used instead of PUI, since formal PUI definitions have only typically been developed during more recent outbreaks such as Severe Acute Respiratory Syndrome (SARS, 2003–2004) [9], Middle East Respiratory Syndrome (MERS, 2012–present) [10], and EVD (during the 2014–2016 West African outbreak) [11].

When new diseases emerge (such as SARS or MERS) or reemerge and new information is learned (such as EVD), a clear and complete clinical description of the disease may not be completely known. Therefore, in such conditions, public health and medical authorities initially develop case definitions to attempt to identify all of the suspect cases in the community according to standardized and current knowledge of the disease. A case definition is a set of uniform criteria used to define a disease for public health surveillance, and the details of the case definition usually form the foundation of the definition of the PUI [8]. Case definitions include the demographic risk factors of persons who may have the disease (age, sex, etc.), the locations where exposure may be occurring, the length of the incubation period of the disease, and the symptoms associated with the disease [12]. A case definition is not equivalent to diagnostic criteria used for a particular disease. Instead, a case definition is intended to ensure maximum sensitivity for disease detection and not necessarily for maximum specificity.

Changes to PUI Definitions during an Outbreak

Maintaining current working knowledge with specific PUI criteria can be extremely challenging for providers, as the case definition may change frequently as new knowledge is learned about the disease. PUI definitions may also be complex and include multiple combinations of risk factors and symptoms to define levels of risk or severity of disease. Symptoms and risk factors may be added to or removed from the formal definition as this process evolves. For example, following two cases of MERS that were diagnosed in healthcare workers from Saudi Arabia traveling to the United States, CDC altered its guidance to emphasize testing for MERS in persons with mild symptoms but with strong epidemiologic risk factors, including particularly prior healthcare exposure [13]. In addition, travel to selected countries or regions may also be included or excluded as a risk factor for disease as an outbreak evolves. During 2015, after the emergence of a nosocomial outbreak of MERS in South Korea, this country was briefly included in the list of countries in the MERS PUI definition and then was subsequently removed when the outbreak ended. When the case definition changes rapidly, information that was recently shared with staff in lectures, webinars, or emails can quickly become obsolete. Unfortunately, it is not uncommon for printed and posted PUI criteria to remain in use long after the content is outdated.

Managing Changes to PUI Definitions

Communicating to Patients

In the setting of evolving PUI definitions, healthcare facilities must focus efforts to encourage patients to identify themselves to staff and to ensure that all those staff who may encounter PUIs have access to the most current information, know how to access that information, and know how to implement necessary actions when a PUI is identified. First, well-placed, clearly written signage in public areas, ambulatory waiting rooms, and ED settings should direct patients to immediately notify specific staff (depending on specific location) if they have either a relevant clinical syndrome (i.e., fever and a cough or fever and a rash) on arrival or if they have traveled internationally during a specified period. The precise time frame for international travel, corresponding to specific infectious incubation periods, will differ based on infection; however a window of travel within the prior 3 weeks will capture the incubation periods of MERS, SARS, novel avian influenza, and EVD and other viral hemorrhagic fevers, which simplifies the message to patients.

Communicating to Facility Staff

Whenever possible, paper or electronic triage forms should be used to prompt staff to ask arriving patients about epidemiologically important risk factors such as travel at each point of entry to the facility and then document the answers prominently in the medical record. However, while prompts can help to increase clinicians' ability to ask about relevant symptoms compatible with HHCD and epidemiologic risk factors (such as travel), it may be challenging for clinicians to remember if the answers they receive from their patients are actually of concern. This is especially true of travel histories, where clinicians may not know which countries are actively affected by outbreaks. Some medical systems have built decision support tools into their electronic medical forms to assist with this challenge and also to guide the subsequent actions a clinician should take whenever a clinical symptom or travel question is answered affirmatively about selected HHCD.

Four Toronto hospitals have described their experience in successfully developing a triage protocol for rapid isolation to limit transmission during the 2003 SARS outbreak [2]. The University of Nebraska ED EVD PUI protocol contains electronic prompts which allow for travel screening completed either by a greeter nurse for walk-in patients or by assigned nurse for patients transported by ambulance services. The travel questions include country of travel and time frame. If the travel screen is positive and the patient has a temperature >101.5 °F, two highly visible alerts appear on the screen, providing specific instructions regarding the immediate next steps including patient isolation and consultation with infectious diseases [14, 15].

Even if decision support tools are not used, providing clinicians with an easily accessible, electronic, expertly maintained list of current infectious diseases of high concern, plus a list, the relevant geographic and other exposure risk factors for each disease can be of tremendous value [16]. Such a list could be curated by hospital infectious diseases or infection prevention staff, local or state public health officials, or others and could be hosted on a local intranet page. Clinical leaders should also consider how they may better direct staff to access expert websites such as that of the CDC, since such sites can sometimes be challenging to navigate for the infrequent user. Quick links built into the electronic medical record (EMR) with bookmarks of relevant internal and/or external website pages related to PUI criteria may be helpful to clinicians and speed their access to relevant information.

In addition to building robust electronic aids into providers' common clinical workflows that can facilitate improving providers' identification of PUIs, it is also essential that frontline clinicians clearly know how to access expert local decision-makers when deciding whether a person meets PUI criteria. Such experts may be infectious disease consultants from the institution where the clinicians work, or a nearby community or tertiary care hospital (if such remote consultation services have been arranged), or may be local or state health department officials. These expert opinions are indispensable to help make the correct determination of whether a patient actually meets PUI criteria.

Maintaining Vigilance

For both patients and staff, in the absence of an ongoing major outbreak during which public attention is highly focused on a specific disease, facilities need to address the challenges of waning interest and vigilance that are likely to occur. During these periods, the continual use of updated signage in public areas, conduct of periodic educational activities, and increasing use of clinical decision support and other types of prompts within the EMR are needed to maintain a consistent level of readiness.

Location of Initial Patient Assessment

PUIs may be identified, and potentially assessed, in several different types of clinical environments.

Telephonic or Remote Triage

The first environment, which is safest for limiting subsequent disease transmission to others, is telephone or Internet triage. Through a remote medical encounter, patients may describe their symptoms to a nurse or other medical provider through a phone conversation, a website questionnaire, or a remote home visit, and it can likely be quickly determined if the patient meets PUI criteria with the required combination of symptoms and exposure risk factors. If the patient does not meet PUI criteria, then his or her triage may be continued as normal. If, however, the patient does meet PUI criteria, then she or he may be directed to a safe portal of entry at an appropriate nearby clinical site for further evaluation and care without unnecessarily exposing other people in a waiting room or other public setting. If EMS is required to help transport the patient to the clinical site, they should be alerted so that they can don the appropriate personal protective equipment (PPE) for transport to limit their own risks of exposure to the disease. In order for this process to be effective, telephone triage staff and providers must have ready access to the most current case definition and PUI criteria.

Ambulatory Triage: Primary or Urgent Care Locations

PUIs may also present in person to a primary care or urgent care office. Primary and urgent care clinics are unlikely to have on-site subject matter expertise in infectious diseases or infection prevention, making the establishment of simple, sustainable protocols essential. These should include (1) use and maintenance of clearly visible signage for arriving patients to instruct them to quickly identify themselves if they have concerning symptoms or risk factors, such as travel, and (2) training of staff who are able to quickly take action (especially including isolation of the patient) should a patient either self-identify with risk factors for an HHCD or be identified as such during triage. In the case of many of the diseases discussed here (MERS, SARS, novel avian influenza), placement in an airborne infection isolation (AII, "negative pressure") room is required as soon as possible. However, since many ambulatory care settings will not have access to AII rooms, in these cases it is recommended to offer the patient a mask, instruct them to put the mask on, and then direct them to a private exam room with a closed door.

After the patient has been safely isolated, senior clinic staff must be notified and must contact appropriate subject matter experts for direction on next steps including (1) whether (based on information already available) the patient meets PUI criteria or if additional information is required; (2) if the latter, direction on the safe use of PPE and distancing from the patient; (3) advice on what types of care can safely be provided in that setting for patients confirmed as PUIs; and (4) instructions on transferring the patient to another more appropriate location for further clinical evaluation and management if deemed necessary.

Emergency Departments

As with primary care and urgent care settings, emergency departments must also be able to identify and isolate patients with infectious diseases, who may arrive as walk-ins, referrals from local primary care or urgent care offices, or by ambulance. Transferring facilities or clinicians should contact the receiving emergency department staff prior to sending a PUI to ensure appropriate isolation space is available, that the patient is immediately taken to the isolation space in a route that is least likely to expose others, and that staff don the appropriate PPE to protect themselves. Further, at the time of transferring a PUI, local public health authorities must be involved in the decision in order to provide expertise as well as logistical and communications support.

Approach

Once the patient has been confirmed to meet PUI criteria and appropriate infectious disease and/or public health experts have been notified, the patient will require transport to an ED capable of fully evaluating the patient (if the patient is not already located in such an ED). For many outpatient practices and clinics, this may be a local ED or perhaps a regional ED. No matter which ED is chosen, it should be assured that they have appropriate plans and resources available to safely clinically evaluate the PUI.

In some regions, the selection of the receiving ED is made jointly between the transferring hospital/clinic and public health officials. In other regions, the decision is left solely to the transferring providers. No matter how the decision process is conducted, protocols for the safe transfer of PUIs to the correct clinical setting must be developed in advance and exercised. This means that primary and urgent care centers should have formal plans for transfer of PUIs to an appropriate ED in their area. In addition, the EMS services and receiving EDs involved in these plans should be fully aware of the plans and their roles within them. Community EDs without the capabilities for evaluating PUIs should have similarly established relationships and plans in place to transfer PUIs to predesignated regional tertiary care centers. EMS must be made aware of the suspected infectious disease when planning a transfer, so that their staff is able to utilize appropriate PPE and other infection control precautions. Receiving hospitals and their surrounding EMS services should meet to review plans for supporting doffing of PPE by EMTs and paramedics, for management of waste generated in transit, and for the procedures to be used to clean the ambulance and return it to service.

While arrangements are being made to transfer the patient, appropriate infection control precautions must be maintained. Personnel should avoid unnecessary contact with the PUI, and all personnel should wear appropriate PPE if they must be near the PUI. Selection of PPE for clinical staff should be selected based on the known (or suspected) routes of transmission for the suspected infection and the resources available. It is not realistic to expect all ambulatory clinics to stock and for staff to maintain proficiency in the correct and consistent use of PPE required in the long-term care of patients for specific infectious diseases such as EVD; however, in the setting of a clinically stable patient, staff should be expected to safely don and doff PPE appropriate for limited patient contact. This may include impermeable gown, N95 respirator, gloves, and face shield. All personnel who wear PPE in this setting must have been previously properly trained to do so.

When the patient is transferred out of the sending facility, the path that EMS personnel will travel out of the clinic should be cleared of other patients, visitors, and other medical personnel to reduce potential exposures. After the patient leaves the facility, the patient care area should be cleaned using preexisting protocols created with input from infection control and public health authorities.

Challenges in Management of the PUI

Depending on the specific infection suspected, the clinical evaluation of the PUI can range from being relatively straightforward to being extraordinarily complex. In 2015, one hospital's experiences in evaluating Ebola virus disease (EVD) PUIs were summarized as the following:

1. Staff was unfamiliar with donning, doffing, and working in personal protective equipment (PPE) appropriate for care of these patients and therefore was apprehensive about their roles.
2. Disproportionate space in clinical areas had to be dedicated exclusively to isolation and care of PUIs, decreasing overall ED capacity.
3. Presence of PUIs in the ED was highly disruptive as the spectacle of cordoned-off spaces and staff in PPE could not be disguised, and large numbers of ancillary personnel congregated in the vicinity of the patient.

4. Patients fearing for their own and family members' safety left the ED waiting area and avoided hospital facilities known to have EVD or PUIs present.
5. The intrusiveness of the media imposed access and flow problems and made it very difficult to protect the identities and protected health information of the PUIs [17].

Other challenges in the evaluation of the PUI have been documented as well. Indeed, during the 2014–2016 EVD outbreak in West Africa, initiation of even basic lab testing and radiologic studies was delayed by 2–3 days in some cases for PUIs in US hospitals, and it was observed that some patients who were PUIs for EVD had poor outcomes because the concern for EVD infection negatively influenced their clinical evaluation and care [18, 19]. Lastly, because the definitive diagnostic tests needed to confirm the presence of HHCD infection may not be available at many hospitals and clinics, and may also take days to confirm or rule out the presence of the suspected infection, the potential period of evaluation for a PUI can extend well beyond a typical clinic or ED visit, further taxing the healthcare system.

Location of Care Delivery

Hospitals must carefully select and prepare the most appropriate location for managing PUIs, ideally well in advance of being asked to care for such a patient. Some hospitals choose to evaluate their PUIs in an ED treatment area, while others use a separate, specialized, inpatient, or other isolation area. When a site within the ED is chosen, there are a few questions that are especially worthy of consideration for planning purposes. First, is the room appropriate to support the care of a patient—is the room AII and is there a private bathroom (or other appropriate individual toileting procedure) available? Second, does the location of the room (or rooms, if multiple rooms will be used) support both safe entry of clean clinical personnel into the room and safe exit for contaminated clinical personnel? Additionally, does the space have a clearly demarcated area for doffing of PPE? One advantageous practice that has been observed is to select a room (or to modify an existing room) that has a separate entrance and exit, so that contaminated staff will not traverse the clean entrance to the room when exiting. Third, is the room in a location within the ED where its use for evaluation of the PUI will not excessively disrupt other ED activities? Evaluation of the PUI can be a labor- and material-intensive process, creating congestion as well as visible distractions for other patients and staff. Therefore, it is advisable, when possible, to choose a room to evaluate PUIs that is located away from the center of the ED to minimize interference to the other important ongoing ED activities and use physical barriers when possible to reduce disruption to routine care. Some facilities plan to keep PUIs in their ED room only until the initial assessment and first round of testing is completed, while other facilities plan to keep their PUIs in the ED room until the diagnosis has been definitively ruled in or out, which can potentially take several days (up to 3 days in the case of EVD).

If it is anticipated that the patient will be required to remain in the room for more than a few hours, plans must consider how both medical waste will safely be removed from the room. Waste management procedures for the PUI must follow the same protocols as for a confirmed patient until the disease is ruled out. If specialized disposal of the waste prior to confirmation of disease is cost-prohibitive for the facility, they must have plans to safely store and secure the waste while awaiting confirmation. One hospital has described the successful use of a portable facility they named a "mobile containment unit" to limit the impact of PUI needs on the main ED while supporting safe patient care [20].

A planning team consisting of an emergency department physician, ED nurse, infectious diseases physician, infection preventionist, facilities manager, and laboratory leadership (at a minimum) should convene to review these questions and begin planning their use of space for PUI evaluation. The team may also wish to explore the utility of video teleconferencing capabilities in the room, which can limit entry to only essential caregivers, allowing others, such as consultants, public health officials, and family members, to remain outside the patient care environment.

Preparation of the Environment of Care

All unnecessary medical equipment and materials should be removed from the room prior to admission of a PUI, leaving only those supplies that will assist with the care and evaluation of the patient. This may include specialized medical equipment, such as a disposable stethoscope or electronic stethoscope, ultrasound machine, or other diagnostic equipment, as well as cleaning supplies and solidification agents for liquid waste if deemed necessary. Biomedical waste receptacles should also be placed in the room. All of the room preparation activities should be guided by the use of predeveloped and exercised checklists, which can ensure that the room and staff are properly prepared to care for the PUI.

Care of the PUI and Establishing a Diagnosis

Once the PUI has arrived in the appropriate clinical location for evaluation, two important parallel processes must begin. The first is to ensure that the patient receives appropriate medical evaluation and care. The second is to undertake the appropriate diagnostic testing to establish a diagnosis. Because the PUI may have immediate medical needs, the receiving clinical facility must be able to provide stabilizing medical care to the patient if necessary, including airway and respiratory support, venous access, and administration of intravenous fluids, parenteral antibiotics, and vasopressor support. The CDC requires that hospitals designated by their states as assessment hospitals for EVD must be able to appropriately manage PUIs, undertaking the necessary diagnostic assays to ensure that other causes of fever (i.e., malaria) are identified and treated in a timely manner [21]. It is important to note that in one hospital's experience, 16% of PUIs who did not ultimately have the HHCD infection suspected did have a life-threatening alternative diagnosis [22].

Receiving facilities must ensure that clinical staff is properly trained to don and doff the necessary PPE in order to provide routine and stabilizing clinical care. In order to do this, hospitals must establish regular training schedules that allow providers to demonstrate proficiency in donning and doffing PPE as well as provide clinical care, manage waste, and obtain laboratory studies according to hospital protocols.

Specialized Care

The range of specific resuscitative and potentially invasive medical services and procedures that will be offered to a PUI before the specific HHCD is ruled out is a highly challenging decision and is one that should be approached carefully. Hospital administrative, medical, legal, and ethical leaders must consider whether they will be able to offer surgical operations (including cesarean sections), hemodialysis, endoscopy, or other procedures that present elevated risks to staff and the facility. These decisions should be made prospectively as part of the hospital planning and preparedness program. If challenging care decisions arise during the care of a specific PUI, an appropriate leadership team should be able to assemble immediately to ensure a fully informed decision-making process. If a specific necessary procedure is not available at the hospital assessing the PUI, public health officials may assist in determining if it may be available elsewhere, such as at one of the ten Regional Ebola and Other Special Pathogen Treatment Centers (RESPTCs) in the United States [10].

Laboratory Testing

Laboratory testing for PUIs may be extremely challenging and requires extensive preplanning in order to support clinical care and establish the diagnosis of specific HHCDs. Prior to the 2014–2016 EVD outbreak, federal guidance stated that all lab testing on patients suspected to have certain highly infectious pathogens (such as EVD) could only be performed in a biosafety level (BSL)-4 laboratory, while most hospitals only have BSL-2 laboratory facilities. Although the CDC provided guidance during the EVD epidemic that was intended to permit appropriate clinical testing outside of BSL-4 labs, these changes were not accepted by many. Many laboratory leaders were concerned about staff safety and impact on use of equipment for routine laboratory studies after processing a sample that could contain EVD [18]. Therefore, clinical and laboratory leaders must jointly decide on the basic menu of laboratory tests to support and to ensure adequate clinical care of the patient with the resources available. Some hospitals have elected to rely on bedside point-of-care testing devices to support much of this need, as the devices eliminate the need to utilize the large, automated laboratory machines. Because malaria is commonly in the differential diagnosis for many PUIs for EVD or other viral hemorrhagic fever, it is important that the hospital have a mechanism for testing for malaria as part of the basic clinical evaluation. To limit the potential spread of biological contamination outside of the patient's room, special procedures must be developed to properly clean and package blood and other biological samples before they leave the room for transport to the hospital lab. Testing for the pathogen of concern is likely to be coordinated through the state public health laboratory. While commercial assays are available for some of these pathogens, public health laboratories will assist in confirmation of the diagnosis or excluding the diagnosis. Hospital staff must be trained and certified in packaging of specimens for transport to state laboratories.

Imaging

Radiographic imaging is an essential component of the evaluation of most febrile patients. Whenever possible, bedside ultrasound is the imaging modality of choice, since it does not require the patient to leave the room and can be interpreted immediately. Portable x-ray imaging can also be used, but may require the use of special protective covers for the machine and the cassette [15]. The decision about whether to offer additional advanced imaging services, such as CT or MRI, depends on variables such as the specific infectivity and transmission of the infectious disease for which the patient is being evaluated. If there is concern about the hospital's ability to offer such imaging services, a multidisciplinary committee, such as the one used to determine the medical and surgical procedures that can be offered, should be utilized.

If the patient is to be transported to an imaging area within the hospital, or to any other area of the hospital, the clinical staff must have a protocol to determine in advance the safest method of doing so. The decision to transport the patient for this purpose should be made by clinical leadership with all relevant parties involved, weighing the risks and benefits of movement of the patient outside of the area of isolation. Hospitals should plan to be able to clear the corridors and elevators of patients, visitors, and others during patient transport when needed and must also have plans in place to decontaminate the transport corridors if necessary following an unintended spill or other event.

Blood Products

The selection and crossmatching of blood products is challenging, because most current practices require use of open blood tubes. Some programs may choose to utilize uncrossmatched type O blood to avoid this risk when transfusion of red blood cells is needed, though others have successfully used a manual slide agglutination test for blood typing as well [15].

Social and Legal Considerations

Hospitals should also plan for special social and legal circumstances that may arise when evaluating the PUI. Hospitals should anticipate how and where they will screen and care for any family members or others who are transported with the PUI to their facility. Hospitals should also consider how they will plan to support the parents and families of pediatric PUIs and whether they can or cannot safely permit family members to stay with a young PUI (or any other PUI) during his or her evaluation [23]. Hospitals should have the ability to utilize language translation services in the area where the PUI assessment occurs. Additionally, hospitals should anticipate how they will respond in the event that a PUI does not wish to comply with the recommended evaluation and/or wants to leave the facility. The University of Nebraska Medical Center has developed a protocol for the noncompliant PUIs [15]. Their protocol was developed following a joint meeting with local law enforcement, public health officials, hospital security, risk management, and ED and hospital leadership.

Preparing for Multiple PUIs

Hospitals should also consider how they will support all of these efforts if they receive more than a single PUI at the same time. Ensuring the availability of appropriate space and trained staff, as well as all of the other tremendous resources required for multiple PUIs, may seem insurmountable but nonetheless requires forethought and planning. Facilities may wish to consider engaging their neighboring hospitals and their public health partners in crafting plans for these efforts.

Conclusions

The use of the identify-isolate-inform framework is essential when patients present to healthcare facilities with symptoms and exposure risk factors of HHCDs. Identification of these patients as early as possible in their presentation, institution of appropriate transmission-based precautions including use of specific PPE and isolation, and prompt notification of relevant experts and authorities are all essential actions in the care for PUIs with HHCDs. Because the potential period of evaluation for a PUI to rule in or rule out disease can extend well beyond a typical clinic or ED visit, thoughtful and coordinated planning efforts are required across the hospital and across the community to be able to adequately care for the PUI.

References

1. Cho SY, Kang JM, Ha YE, Park GE, Lee JY, Ko JH, et al. MERS-CoV outbreak following a single patient exposure in an emergency room in South Korea: an epidemiological outbreak study. Lancet (London, England). 2016;388(10048):994–1001.
2. Borgundvaag B, Ovens H, Goldman B, Schull M, Rutledge T, Boutis K, et al. SARS outbreak in the greater Toronto area: the emergency department experience. CMAJ. 2004;171(11):1342–4.
3. Liu JW, Lu SN, Chen SS, Yang KD, Lin MC, Wu CC, et al. Epidemiologic study and containment of a nosocomial outbreak of severe acute respiratory syndrome in a medical center in Kaohsiung, Taiwan. Infect Control Hosp Epidemiol. 2006;27(5):466–72.
4. Teleman MD, Boudville IC, Heng BH, Zhu D, Leo YS. Factors associated with transmission of severe acute respiratory syndrome among health-care workers in Singapore. Epidemiol Infect. 2004;132(5):797–803.
5. Chevalier MS, Chung W, Smith J, Weil LM, Hughes SM, Joyner SN, et al. Ebola virus disease cluster in the United States--Dallas County, Texas, 2014. MMWR Morb Mortal Wkly Rep. 2014;63(46):1087–8.
6. Chung WM, Smith JC, Weil LM, Hughes SM, Joyner SN, Hall EM, et al. Active tracing and monitoring of contacts associated with the first cluster of Ebola in the United States. Ann Intern Med. 2015;163(3):164–73.
7. Chea N, Perz J, Srinivasan A, Laufer A, et al. Identify, isolate, inform: background and considerations for Ebola virus disease preparedness in U.S. ambulatory care settings. Am J Infect Control. 2015;43(11):1244–5.
8. Centers for Disease Control and Prevention. Key terms used in case classifications: Centers for Disease Control and Prevention; 2015 [updated December 17, 2015. Available from: https://wwwn.cdc.gov/nndss/terms.html.
9. Centers for Disease Control and Prevention. Clinical guidance on the identification and evaluation of possible SARS-CoV disease among persons presenting with community-acquired illness (version 2): Centers for Disease Control and Prevention; 2012 [updated July 7, 2012. Available from: https://www.cdc.gov/sars/clinical/guidance.html.
10. Centers for Disease Control and Prevention. Interim patient under investigation (PUI) guidance and case definitions: Centers for Disease Control and Prevention; 2016 [updated July 13, 2016. Available from: https://www.cdc.gov/coronavirus/mers/case-def.html.
11. Centers for Disease Control and Prevention. Case definition for Ebola virus disease (EVD): Centers for Disease Control and Prevention; 2016 [updated November 16, 2014. Available from: https://www.cdc.gov/vhf/ebola/healthcare-us/evaluating-patients/case-definition.html.
12. Centers for Disease Control and Prevention. Outbreak case definitions: Centers for Disease Control and Prevention; 2016 [updated May 5, 2016. Available from: https://www.cdc.gov/urdo/downloads/casedefinitions.pdf.
13. Schneider E, Chommanard C, Rudd J, Whitaker B, Lowe L, Gerber SI. Evaluation of patients under investigation for MERS-CoV infection, United States, January 2013–October 2014. Emerg Infect Dis. 2015;21(7):1220–3.
14. Schwedhelm S, Msn RN, Swanhorst J, Bsn RN, Watson S, Bsn RN, et al. ED Ebola triage algorithm: a tool and process for compliance. J Emerg Nurs. 2015;41(2):165–9.
15. Wadman MC, Schwedhelm SS, Watson S, Swanhorst J, Gibbs SG, Lowe JJ, et al. Emergency department processes for the evaluation and management of persons under investigation for Ebola virus disease. Ann Emerg Med. 2015;66(3):306–14.
16. Le A, Biddinger P, Smith P, Herstein J, Levy D, Gibbs S, et al. A highly infectious disease care network within the United States healthcare system. Health Secur. 2017;15(3):282–7.
17. Bogucki S, Isakov A. Patients under investigation for Ebola virus disease in the United States: hospital preparedness planning and alternate care facilities. Acad Emerg Med. 2015;22(5):600–4.

18. Van Beneden CA, Pietz H, Kirkcaldy RD, Koonin LM, Uyeki TM, Oster AM, et al. Early identification and prevention of the spread of Ebola - United States. MMWR Suppl. 2016;65(3):75–84.
19. Karwowski MP, Meites E, Fullerton KE, Stroher U, Lowe L, Rayfield M, et al. Clinical inquiries regarding Ebola virus disease received by CDC–United States, July 9–November 15, 2014. MMWR Morb Mortal Wkly Rep. 2014;63(49):1175–9.
20. Sugalski G, Murano T, Fox A, Rosania A. Development and use of mobile containment units for the evaluation and treatment of potential Ebola virus disease patients in a United States hospital. Acad Emerg Med. 2015;22(5):616–22.
21. Jeon MH, Kim TH. Institutional preparedness to prevent future Middle East respiratory syndrome coronavirus-like outbreaks in Republic of Korea. Infect Chemother. 2016;48(2):75–80.
22. Fairley JK, Kozarsky PE, Kraft CS, Guarner J, Steinberg JP, Anderson E, et al. Ebola or not? Evaluating the ill traveler from Ebola-affected countries in West Africa. Open Forum Infect Dis. 2016;3(1):ofw005.
23. Davies HD, Byington CL, Committee on Infectious Diesease. Parental presence during treatment of Ebola or other highly consequential infection. Pediatrics. 2016;138(3):e20161891.

Maintenance of Preparedness 13

Timo Wolf

Introduction

Although outbreaks of highly hazardous communicable diseases (HHCD) that require patients to be cared for in a high-level isolation unit (HLIU) can occur at any time, we have seen distinct periods with public health emergencies of international concern that created huge challenges to medical systems throughout many parts of the world, most notably the Ebola crisis in 2014 and the SARS epidemic in 2003. These crises led to an upscaling of isolation capacities in many countries and have also influenced the design of HLIUs as well as our thinking of how advanced the level of care provided under isolation conditions can or should be. Many units in the 1960s and 1970s were essentially conceived with a focus on containment, with comparatively few possibilities of medical care provision [1]. The SARS epidemic produced a dramatic need to provide critical care and ventilatory support under safe conditions in order to avoid transmission of infection to intensive care staff [2], and in the 2014–2016 Ebola outbreak, patients treated in the USA and Europe frequently required intensive care procedures inclusive of ventilatory support and renal replacement therapy [3]. Many of these procedures were performed for the first time in the setting of isolation precautions, even at the few specialized centers that exist. Although diseases like Lassa have sporadically produced import cases of hemorrhagic fevers in Europe and the USA [4], public health emergencies of international concern were generally followed by intervals of many years in which there were few or no cases. Hence, one of the challenges for many HLIUs is to maintain the capability to provide high-level care under isolation conditions in these intervals, which are long enough to undergo considerable staff fluctuation and changes in therapeutic algorithms and technology. Moreover, medical advances that occur in the meantime

T. Wolf (✉)
Department of Infectious Diseases, University Hospital,
Theodor Stern Kai 7, Frankfurt 60596, Germany
e-mail: Timo.wolf@kgu.de

A. Hewlett, A. R. K. Murthy (eds.), *Bioemergency Planning*,
https://doi.org/10.1007/978-3-319-77032-1_13

have to be translated into the setting of isolation treatment without the chance to realistically test them under these conditions. Additionally, the provision of high-level isolation medical care requires complicated standards and procedures that can easily be forgotten in "peacetime". It is thus of crucial importance to maintain a certain level of preparedness over extended periods of time until the next emergency occurs, necessitating HLIUs to be prepared to begin operations very quickly.

> "You can plan events, but if they go according to your plan, they are not events."
>
> John Berger, 1926

At the end of the day, however, we should realize that we have to be prepared for new circumstances, sometimes for even the unplannable. We have to be aware that the management of biological hazards requires a great deal of flexibility.

Infrastructure

HLIUs are part of the critical infrastructure required to react to biological hazards, may they be individual cases of highly contagious diseases, public health emergencies of international concern or the deliberate release of biological agents. HLIUs provide levels of infection control for healthcare workers and the community that cannot easily be provided in another setting. This level of infection control is necessary for HHCDs like Ebola, Lassa, SARS, Crimean-Congo hemorrhagic fever, smallpox and many others but may also be needed in case of new biological hazards of which the impact is yet unknown. There are different plans on the national level concerning the number of HLIUs required to maintain preparedness. Germany, the UK, the USA and Sweden, for example, possess more than one HLIU; however, other countries may have just one HLIU or even just a care agreement with neighboring countries [5]. The advantages of having more than one unit include shorter, safer journeys for patients from the referral point to the unit, cross-covering between units (e.g. when one unit is closed for maintenance), and the potential for a broader range of specialists. The number of staff needed for the treatment of an individual case can become massive if the patient condition requires very intensive treatment [6], and the availability of staff from a unit nearby may provide relief. This however requires coordination in skill maintenance and training, so that healthcare professionals can easily adapt to the local procedures and infrastructure within another unit. Disadvantages include increased costs, less frequent use and dispersion of clinical expertise. It is thus important to adapt the maintenance preparations to the network that an HLIU or a regional hospital is integrated into.

Another aspect of the planning of maintenance is how many patients an individual HLIU would be expected to care for. Even an individual imported case of a disease of high consequence may have contact cases that need to be admitted in case of the development of symptoms. These contact patients may be cared for in separate units but may also be concentrated in one unit, depending on the local procedures. An individual case of a hemorrhagic fever would usually produce very few contact cases, but respiratory pathogens of high consequence may produce many contact cases, particularly if the exposure occurs within an aircraft, leaving many contact patients with no place to go to where they can be monitored for symptoms of infection.

When planning for an event, it is always important to consider that should such an event occur, it will be necessary to maintain operational and business continuity. Essentially, in the context of a larger hospital, this means that for critical infrastructure areas such as ICUs, ERs, radiology and others that may not be overtly affected, the care of remaining patients should be maintained at an acceptable level. This will mean that staff must not be overly exhausted to a point where staff shortage will be created before or after the event.

The infrastructure utilized will require regular maintenance on a technical level. Waste disposal systems, ventilation systems, decontamination systems, machinery-like point-of-care diagnostics, ventilators, dialysis machines and many more items will require regular use, maintenance and possibly repair. It will become necessary to have technicians and medical professionals perform this in regular intervals, sometimes as short as weekly. This is a crucial amount of work that is often underestimated.

Supply Maintenance

One very fundamental question is what supplies and medications need to be stockpiled prior to event occurrence. It is impossible to give a universal recommendation on what type and how much of each material or medication will be required, as this depends on very individual circumstances. The precise type of personal protective equipment (PPE) used can greatly influence the necessary quantities. For example, some respirator suits use overalls with integrated gloves and some without. When using integrated gloves, the sizes of the complete suits available at an individual center must be very diverse, as a bad fit of a glove can be a safety hazard. Thus, complete suits must be available in all sizes to ensure proper fit. This means that the stockpiling will require larger quantities for the integrated models. Furthermore, the life span of a glove is much shorter than the one of the suit material, so that for the same amount of time, more suits will be needed based on the life span for the integrated model. Suits with no integrated gloves may be stockpiled in fewer size models, and gloves can be ordered separately. It is also important to be aware of what parts of the PPE are reusable and what parts will be discarded after use. Reusable material does not require stockpiling but does require regular function tests. It is extremely helpful to have experience with the amount of a particular type of PPE used in a real case in order to determine on how much stockpiling is needed.

It is economical to keep stockpiling to the absolute minimum necessary and to avoid discarding unused material. Most of the stockpiled material can be used for training purposes. It must be kept in mind, however, that in the situation of a public health emergency, the demand for PPE and other material required may drastically rise [8] and outnumber the production capacity of the various producers. Therefore, the most critical infrastructure must maintain a safety margin of 3–4 weeks demand of material. Although it may be wise to harmonize the material used in adjacent HLIUs, as this would facilitate cross coverage if available, this may create issues with availability if too many HLIUs are using material by the same supplier.

Most of the diseases that HLIUs will deal with are orphan diseases, for which standard treatment is not available. However, it is helpful to think of substances that could be available for treatment. In some countries, health authorities may keep a supply of orphan drugs or of experimental medication. The CDC and the Public Health Agency of Canada maintain such supplies. Other countries like Germany do not maintain these supplies on a national level and leave this to individual HLIUs and local health authorities. Consideration should be given to maintaining a supply of ribavirin, which has proven useful for the treatment of Lassa as well as RSV pneumonitis in addition to its licenced indication for treatment of hepatitis C. However, particularly for Lassa fever, it should be administered intravenously, and the intravenous formulation may be difficult to obtain. It may also be helpful to have access to vaccines that can be used as a post-exposure prophylaxis, such as the rVSV Ebola virus vaccine [9].

Staff Training

One of the most important and demanding tasks for managers of HLIUs is to have adequate staff from different specialties readily available and capable of providing specialized HLIU patient care. The number of physicians, nurses and other health professionals required rises with the severity of the disease in question. For example, in the Frankfurt HLIU, 88 staff members were involved in the treatment of one Ebola patient [6]. Similarly, the Nebraska Biocontainment Unit and the Emory Serious Communicable Diseases Unit utilized 5–6 and 2–3 nursing staff members per shift, respectively, when caring for Ebola patients [7]. When intensive care and specialized treatments are utilized, certain tasks may not be able to be performed by the core nursing and physician team. Whilst renal replacement therapy and minor technical questions can easily be handled by experienced ICU staff, more difficult questions may necessitate other specialized staff within the unit. Transfusion management, radiology and processing of laboratory specimens may be accomplished by specialists that are trained to enter the unit. Depending on the training of the physicians on the core team, procedures like endoscopy and surgery may require a specialist to enter the unit as well. Many HLIUs also train pediatric and obstetric nurses and physicians in order to ensure a high level of care for children and pregnant women. As an example, Table 13.1 demonstrates an annual training schedule used in the Frankfurt HLIU (Figs. 13.1, 13.2 and 13.3).

Time must be allocated for training staff and for regular maintenance testing of specialized systems. The frequency of training and maintenance is decided by local and technical requirements. A formalized contract will often be needed to maintain these functions. The training is oriented towards an effective standard operating procedure to evacuate any current patients from the unit and to prepare the HLIU for

Table 13.1 Exercise schedule as used in the Frankfurt HLIU

Topic	Required	Duration	I	II	III	IV	V	VI	VII	VIII	IX	X	XI	XII
Education meeting/general information	Once yearly	90 min			X							X		
Drill with other HLIU	Once yearly	6 h	X											
Drill for ICU staff in the HLIU	Every second year	7 h		X										
Educational meeting on viral hemorrhagic fevers	Once yearly	2 h			X			X						
Alarm chain and preparation of HLIU	Once yearly	2 h	X		X								X	
Use of PPE and isolation procedure	Four times yearly	3.5 h	Every second week											
Technical training and waste disposal	Twice yearly	3.5 h		X		X				X				
Emergencies and CPR under isolation conditions	Twice yearly	3.5 h		X		X							X	
Dangerous goods and material shipping	Every second year	1 h									X			

Roman numerals stand for months

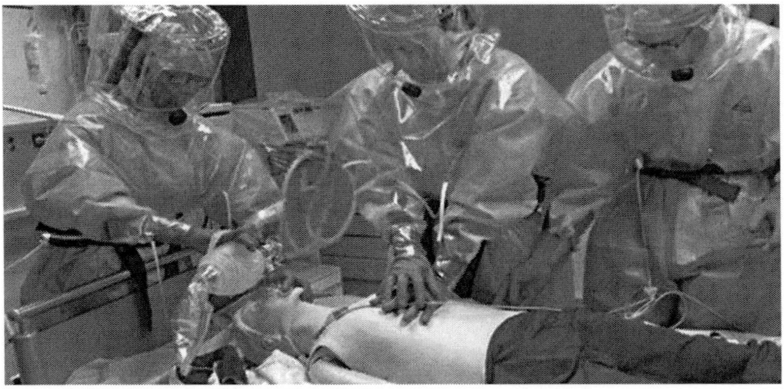

Fig. 13.1 Life support training for HLIU staff. Due to limited communication, algorithms for emergencies need to be practiced frequently. Ideally, team members will be able to go through algorithms with very little verbal communication.

Fig. 13.2 Staff member of the Frankfurt HLIU team practicing intravenous techniques while in PPE. The placement of intravenous catheters is more demanding due to the lack of sensitivity in thick gloves. Thorough training needs to be performed in order to avoid needlestick injuries.

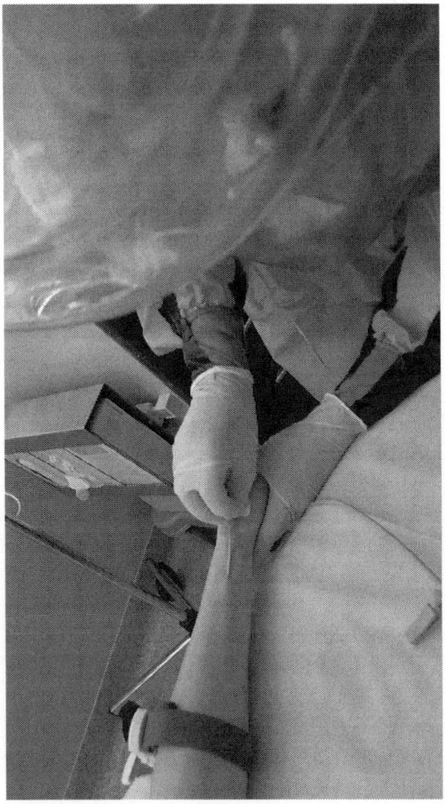

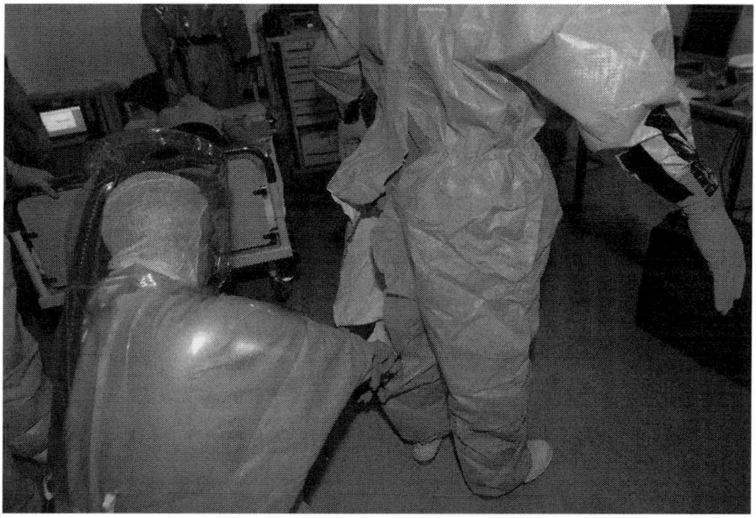

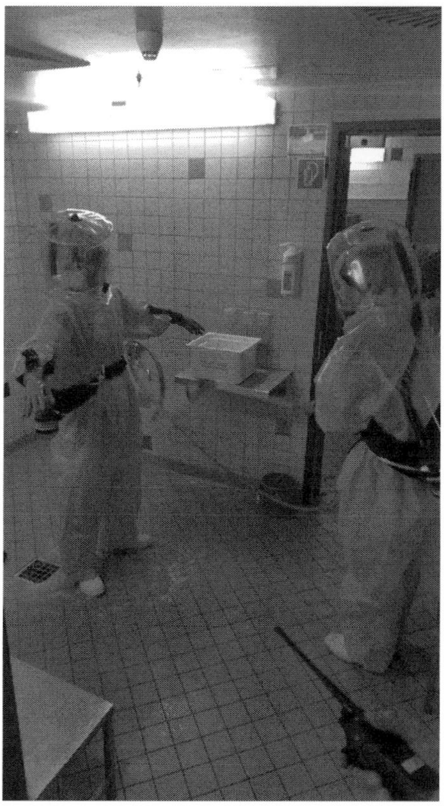

Fig. 13.3 The PPE doffing and decontamination process is crucial and bears a higher contamination risk, so practicing this skill is an important part of HLIU maintence of preparedness programs. Some units may therefore utilize a buddy system, where doffing and decontamination is performed with the assistance of a second staff member in order to avoid mistakes

admission of a patient with a highly hazardous communicable disease within a designated amount of time without compromising patient care. This amount of time is decided by local requirements. For the Frankfurt HLIU, which is only 15 min away from a major international airport, this period is naturally very short. It might be preferable to admit non-HHCD patients to an HLIU only when other isolation facilities are not available and to transfer these patients from the HLIU as soon as practical. On the other hand, regular use of the HLIU facilitates the regular maintenance of systems. The HLIU is however not the only unit involved in maintenance of preparedness training. Procedures need also to be practiced with local emergency departments, emergency medical services, the local health authorities and the reference, high-level security laboratories to provide for safe intersections of announcing and transporting patients and patient material.

Some units have shared their curricula in order to provide information on the content of maintenance of preparedness training [10]. This content provides a minimum threshold of theoretical knowledge and practical skills necessary to safely treat a patient with a suspected or confirmed HHCD. Maintenance of preparedness training should consist of the following:

- Identifying patients with suspected diseases of high consequence
- Disease-specific knowledge, including epidemiology and public health response
- Infection control, including the correct use of personal protective equipment (PPE), decontamination and the safe management of clinical waste
- Providing healthcare in the setting of a high-level isolation unit
- The use of specialized medical devices and equipment (e.g. patient isolators, respirators) found in this setting
- The medical management of contact patients

Other important aspects of preparedness include:

- Bio-security, including safe transport of specimens and safe patient transfer
- Crisis management and crisis communication
- Regular exercises for patient care teams

These recommendations were mainly influenced by the experience of the SARS epidemic. However, during the 2014–2016 Ebola outbreak, the level of care provided and necessary in the treatment of patients was quite different from the experience with SARS. It was formerly thought that procedures like ventilation, renal replacement therapy and CPR would be too risky in the care of a hemorrhagic fever patient, and there was no evidence to support its use. Based on the experience of treating Ebola patients in resource-rich countries, and later also in the endemic area in Western Africa, this limited approach was reconsidered and revised. It was shown that the provision of modern intensive care medicine was possible and successful [11, 12].

Patients with HHCDs may require a range of interventions, including transfusion of blood/blood products; cardiac, respiratory and invasive hemodynamic monitoring; radiography; ultrasonography; minor surgical procedures (e.g. thoracocentesis); renal dialysis; and mechanical ventilation. The input from critical care clinicians is essential to patient management. There is guidance on the application of the most complicated procedures, e.g. for renal replacement therapy (RRT) [13]. This may provide some orientation on which modality of RRT, choice of anticoagulation and PPE is used in conjunction with this method, as well as on the disinfection and decontamination questions that arise in this context. It can be anticipated that the guidelines on the provision of care to patients with HHCDs will constantly evolve and continue to improve.

HLIUs should therefore be equipped to provide the level of care available in an intensive care unit, and critical care clinicians should routinely train alongside the HLIU team. Support from other specialties (e.g. nephrology, pediatrics, cardiology, obstetrics) may also be necessary, so specialist clinicians should be pre-identified and train alongside the HLIU team. Additionally, needs for specialist non-clinical expertise (e.g. to repair ventilation systems or maintain near-patient testing equipment) should be assessed, and relevant staff trained appropriately in advance. Partly trained or newly trained individuals who need to enter the unit should be given just-in-time training, be escorted and be fully supervised. Ideally, psychological support should also be offered to the participants of an HLIU team, so it is important to include specialists in this area in ongoing maintenance of preparedness efforts.

Occupational Health and Safety

The occupational health department needs to be closely associated with the HLIU in order to ensure safety for staff of HLIU. In some countries, there are regulations for personnel who work in respirators or hoods, including pulmonary function testing. Even if not required, it is important to discuss respiratory health with healthcare workers willing to participate in HLIU treatment. The occupational health department can also assist with providing and maintining records on vaccination and respiratory fit testing for HLIU team members.

It is very important to be aware that some staff will have or may develop anxieties when working with patients with HHCDs, and the occupational health department should work with behavioral health specialists to assist healthcare workers in the HLIU environment. (see Chap. 16) These anxieties may not be apparent in the early stages of training and may arise only when confronted with a "real" situation. It is an important aspect of preparedness to address potential or already existing anxieties, keeping in mind that the expression of fear does not mean that a staff member can no longer work in an HLIU. It rather means that he or she should receive information on the following:

- Facts about biological hazards
- Detailed facts about the transmissibility of a disease

- How healthcare workers can protect themselves most efficiently
- Guidelines on how to care for HHCD patients
- Measures to avoid the spread of pathogens

Along with fear of the disease itself, healthcare workers may also have anxiety stemming from concern that patients cannot be adequately taken care of in the HLIU setting and that individual standards of care cannot be met, placing the patients at a disadvantage. These anxieties can be mitigated through education and discussion with a behavioral health provider.

It is very important to maintain a strong level of team building and trust within the HLIU staff to enhance safety. Preparedness does not only necessitate regular education and skills building but also a good knowledge of the professional capabilities of each team member. Team building events held within or outside of the work environment can facilitate ongoing relationships between members of the team when the HLIU is not activated and serve to enhance preparedness through maintenance of trust within the team [14].

Coordination

Maintaining the functionality of a HLIU requires working in line with other units and professions. Very crucial areas of collaboration that necessitate ongoing coordination are the transport and receiving process of patients. Establishing and maintaining relationships with local emergency medical services is crucial to preparedness, as discussed in the Transport chapter of this text.

It is also possible that a patient with a HHCD will arrive at the emergency department contained within the facility where the HLIU is located. This requires that a team of experts should be ready to organize and establish isolation capacity quickly; thus emergency department personnel should be incorporated into the HLIU maintenance of preparedness schedule on a regular basis.

Most HLIUs rely on reference laboratories that are experienced in the diagnosis of special pathogens. The coordination between laboratory and the HLIU is another focal point of preparedness activities in peacetime. It can be a very demanding task to organize the transport of material to the laboratory, as there are regulations and safety measures to adhere to. There are commercial courier companies that are capable of transporting specimens potentially containing special pathogens, and these relationships should be pre-established. In all cases, the transport of material to the laboratory and an emergency plan for exposed laboratory workers need to be practised and prepared.

Conclusion

Necessities in the Maintenance of Preparedness

- A designated clinical leader
- A designated nurse leader
- Successors for both positions and deputies in case of unavailability
- An HLIU-specific training program with standardized curricula with an accurate recording and documentation system for attendance
- 24/7 availability system to open the unit at the shortest possible notice
- A standard procedure for becoming operational when activated
- A staff roster allowing full coverage as needed within a minimum amount of time
- Regular emergency and evacuation training
- Regular maintenance of medical machinery (POCT diagnostics, ventilators, RRT machines, etc.)
- Regular maintenance and testing of communication systems and camera systems for monitoring the unit from outside
- Regular testing of negative pressure ventilation system and waste disposal system
- Regular training of standard procedures of HLIU treatment provision
- Updating of staff lists necessary for care
- Adaptation of PPE, medical machinery and communication systems to latest standards
- Occupational health maintenance of HLIU team (vaccines, respiratory fit testing, behavioral health, etc.)
- Regular education about emerging infectious diseases and current challenges or outbreaks

The management of HHCDs requires the maintenance of a satisfactory level of preparedness. In order to maintain this preparedness, it is important to have a precise plan on how an individual HLIU is operational in the framework of local, regional and national plans. The maximum number of patients that would be admitted, the level of care provided within the HLIU and the technical prerequisites of the unit determines what measures need to be taken. One of the most important aspects of preparedness is the ability to maintain adequate numbers of trained staff capable of safely working in an HLIU. It is helpful to have protocols that provide guidance for nurses, physicians and others, as well as for the number of staff that need to be included in the training. The materials and supplies required depend on the type of PPE, equipment used and the size of the team. It is important to have a good understanding of the number of supplies that are required for the treatment of a real case in order to inform decisions on stockpiling necessary supplies. Training requirements are substantial, and adequate time must be provided to accomplish this. The psychological burden of working on an HLIU should be respected, and staff should receive information, counselling and team building measures to reduce that burden. These measures to maintain preparedness need to be well integrated and coordinated with interfaces like reference laboratories, transport organizations and the surrounding hospital infrastructure. Taken together, these measures will enable HLIUs to be ready when they are needed and are investments of time and resources that are necessary, even in the temporal absence of HHCD cases.

References

1. Kortepeter MG, Kwon EH, Hewlett AL, Smith PW, Cieslak TJ. Containment care units for managing patients with highly hazardous infectious diseases: a concept whose time has come. J Inf Dis. 2016;214(S3):S137–41.
2. Loeb M, McGeer A, Henry B, Ofner M, et al. SARS among critical care nurses, Toronto. Emerg Infect Dis [serial online], 10(2). Available at https://wwwnc.cdc.gov/eid/article/10/2/03-0838_article.
3. Uyeki T, Mehta AK, Davey RT Jr, Liddell AM, et al. Working Group of the U.S.–European clinical network on clinical management of Ebola virus disease patients in the U.S. and Europe. Clinical management of Ebola virus disease in the United States and Europe. N Engl J Med. 2016;374(7):636–46.
4. European Center for Disease Prevention. Rapid risk assessment – Lassa fever in Nigeria, Benin, Togo, Germany and USA. http://ecdc.europa.eu/en/publications/Publications/RRA-Lassa-fever-Germany-march-2016.pdf. Accessed 3 May 2017.
5. Bannister B, Puro V, Fusco FM, Heptonstall J, Ippolito G, for the EUNID Working Group. Framework for the design and operation of high-level isolation units: consensus of the European network of infectious diseases. Lancet Infect Dis. 2009;9:45–56.
6. Zacharowski K, Brodt HR, Wolf T. Medical treatment of an Ebola-infected doctor–ethics over costs? Lancet. 2015;385(9969):685.
7. Hewlett A, Vasa A, Cieslak TJ, Lowe J, Schwedhelm M. Viral hemorrhagic fever preparedness. In: Bearman M-P, Morgan M, editors. Infection prevention: new perspectives and controversies. New York: Springer. [In Press].
8. Abutaleb Y for Reuters. U.S. Ebola fears fuel new demand for protective gear. October 14, 2014. Online at https://www.yahoo.com/news/u-ebola-fears-fuel-demand-protective-gear-234506969--sector.html. Accessed 13 May 2017.
9. Lai L, Davey R, Beck A, Xu Y, et al. Emergency postexposure vaccination with vesicular stomatitis virus-vectored Ebola vaccine after needlestick. JAMA. 2015;313(12):1249–55.
10. Baka A, Fusco FM, Puro V, et al. A curriculum for training healthcare workers in the management of highly infectious diseases. Euro Surveill. 2007;12(6):A3.
11. Murthy S, on behalf of the Ebola Clinical Care authors group. Ebola and provision of critical care. Lancet. 2015;385:1392–3.
12. Wolf T, Kann G, Becker S, et al. Severe Ebola virus disease with vascular leakage and multiorgan failure: treatment of a patient in intensive care. Lancet. 2014; published online Dec 19. https://doi.org/10.1016/S0140-6736(14)62384-9.
13. Wolf T, Ross MJ, Davenport A. Minimizing risks associated with renal replacement therapy in patients with Ebola virus disease. Kidney Int. 2015;87:5–7.
14. Smith PW, Boulter KC, Hewlett AL, et al. Planning and response to Ebola virus disease: an integrated approach. Am J Infect Control. 2015;43(5):441–6. https://doi.org/10.1016/j.ajic.2015.01.019.

14 Personal Protective Equipment

Jill S. Morgan

Key Terms

PPE	Personal protective equipment, specifically that worn or used by healthcare providers during patient care
HCW	Healthcare worker, may be physician, nurse, therapist, or laboratorian
Impervious	Resistant to penetration by liquids and small particles
Don(ning)	Putting on, as in gloves or clothing
Doff(ing)	Removing gloves or clothing
PAPR	Powered air-purifying respirators
ABHR	Alcohol-based hand rubs
Trained Observer	A person familiar with procedures and protocols, especially donning and doffing, whose role is to watch other staff for compliance while they perform those procedures
Aerosol generating	Procedures or acts that may produce very small droplets of body fluids
Proprioception	Awareness of where our body is in space
Mindfulness	Focusing one's attention at the present, being aware of one's situation and surroundings
Inoculation	The introduction of a microorganism into a person or organism

J. S. Morgan (✉)
Serious Communicable Disease Unit, Emory University Hospital, Atlanta, GA, USA
e-mail: jill.morgan@emoryhealthcare.org

A. Hewlett, A. R. K. Murthy (eds.), *Bioemergency Planning*,
https://doi.org/10.1007/978-3-319-77032-1_14

Introduction

Mindfulness may not be a term usually associated with personal protective equipment (PPE), but it is a useful concept for the discussion of putting together, layer by layer, the protective barriers that allow the safe provision of care for patients with highly hazardous communicable diseases. Each piece of the full PPE ensemble will have limitations that must be understood by the wearer. Close and careful attention to behaviors in the patient care environment becomes good PPE etiquette. Donning, or putting on PPE, carefully and fully before attending to a patient's needs is fundamental but not intuitive. Doffing, or removing PPE, is a high-risk procedure that can be performed safely with practice, coaching, and observation. Mitigating risk depends on awareness to all areas of potential contamination and a mindful approach to delivering safe patient care.

The recommendations concerning PPE for healthcare workers (HCWs) have evolved in fits and starts, frequently prompted by outbreaks, such as severe acute respiratory syndrome (SARS), and emerging pathogens, such as HIV. It is inconceivable to many current healthcare workers that disposable glove use was neither mandatory nor recommended until the 1970s [1]. The recommendations for isolation, PPE use, and hand hygiene have continued to change as recently as the Ebola virus disease (EVD) outbreak of 2014–2016.

From the time it was recognized that germs could cause disease, ways to avoid those germs have been sought. Barrier methods, including early gloves made of sheep intestines, were the beginning of personal protective devices aimed to provide a boundary isolating the healthcare provider from some aspect of the patient thought to be infected, such as a wound [2]. Isolating patients is another means of separating HCWs from potentially infectious patients. As the understanding of pathogens and transmissibility has evolved, so has the use of isolation and barriers for protection.

The categories for isolation correspond to the type or portion of a patient that requires some barrier method, for instance, gloves for wound care in the 1970s become gloves for all blood and bodily fluids by the 1980s (Table 14.1).

Patients themselves are not the only source of risk for healthcare workers. As early as the 1500s, it was recognized that surfaces and materials that had contact with patients or their body fluids could also serve to spread disease from patient to patient and from patient to staff [3]. A fomite is any article or surface that can harbor pathogens. The length of time a pathogen can remain viable on such surfaces is highly variable, from minutes to hours and days. All surfaces within the patient care environment, including bed linens, walls, and floors, can be potential sources for contamination.

The method by which a person is inoculated inadvertently by a pathogen can be either through direct or indirect contact. Direct inoculation occurs when infective blood or body substance comes in contact with another person's mucous membranes or broken skin. Indirect inoculation occurs when contact is first made with a contaminated intermediary and then into the eyes, nose, mouth, or non-intact skin [1]. The goal of all PPE is to prevent direct inoculation. Adherence to PPE etiquette and a doffing protocol serves to minimize the potential for indirect inoculation.

Table 14.1 Changes in US isolation precaution recommendations [1]

1970	1983	1988	1996
Infectious disease specialty hospitals and TB facilities closed, moving these patients into the general population. Categories of isolation include:	Category or disease specific as chosen by facility. Categories of isolation include:	Universal precautions: Blood and bodily fluids containing visible blood, of all patients. Did not apply to non-bloody feces, nasal secretions, sputum, sweat, tears, or urine	Standard precautions include blood and bodily fluid for all plus transmission-based precautions which include:
Strict	Strict		Airborne
Respiratory	Respiratory		Contact
Protective	TB		Droplet
Enteric	Contact		
Wound/skin	Drainage/secretion		
Discharge	Blood/body fluid		
Blood			
PPE recommendations			
Disposable gloves, new in mid-1960s, for use with known infectious substances	Up to HCWs to decide likelihood of contamination and use gown, glove, mask if indicated by risk for known or suspected infected materials	Gloves for contact with blood or bodily fluids. Hand washing recommended after all glove removal. Masks and protective eyewear for procedures with splash risk, all patients	PPE for contact with blood and certain bodily fluids considered potentially infectious. Still excepted: feces, sputum, sweat, tears, urine, and vomitus unless blood is visible

Protective equipment, from the early gloves to N95 masks and new impervious surface gowns, has become a routine part of working inside western healthcare facilities. It is easy to assume that what is common is also simple and that assumption has been extended to PPE use. It is common in the hospital setting to assume healthcare workers are proficient in all aspects of PPE. The use of PPE by healthcare workers came under scrutiny during the West African outbreak of EVD in 2014–2016. Concerns were raised about the readiness to treat patients with highly hazardous communicable diseases within US hospitals [4]. While caring for patients in isolation is something that US healthcare workers do every day, that familiarity does not assure competency.

Multiple studies conducted before and since the Ebola outbreak confirm that contamination to the wearer can occur even with careful use of PPE [5, 6]. While healthcare workers may believe that adding more layers and items to their PPE ensemble increases their safety, this has not been demonstrated to be true [7]. In caring for patients with highly hazardous communicable diseases, risks are mitigated with information about disease transmission, the choice of the right PPE ensemble, training and practice, and the use of trained observers. The margin for error is small inside biocontainment units. It must be recognized by all team members that violations of infection control protocols, including PPE use and etiquette, can negate the compliant work of others and put everyone at risk [8].

In examining the makeup of a PPE ensemble, the advantages and the liabilities of each piece will be examined. PPE etiquette, or good form, will be evaluated, from the donning of PPE through its use at the bedside to the importance of a safe and observed doffing procedure.

The CDC has issued guidelines for the PPE to be worn by healthcare workers in the care and treatment of Ebola patients, guidelines that were updated frequently during the outbreak [9]. Those guidelines, and the choices of PPE made by the hospitals that cared successfully for patients with Ebola, reflect the need for total body coverage, including respiratory protection. While Ebola virus disease is not generally considered an airborne disease, the care of these patients may keep healthcare workers in close proximity to patients for extended periods of time and require them to perform tasks and procedures that generate aerosols; thus, respiratory protection is warranted.

The choice of a PPE ensemble is dependent upon other previous decisions, many of which are made far from the bedside. Ultimately, the PPE that is worn by staff is made up of items that can be sourced reliably and affordably, complies with all safety regulations, and in which the staff have competency in using through regular training and education. Deciding on one uniform type of PPE is also dependent on facility design and work flow. Below is list of questions to consider that may affect the choice of PPE and the protocols for its use. These questions can help guide the formation of a PPE matrix ensuring that all staff are protected commensurate with their level of risk. All personnel who come in direct contact with the patient; patient belongings; patient waste, including packaged waste; as well as the patient's direct environment must use appropriate PPE and be trained in its use [10].

- Will all staff wear the same PPE?
- Where will staff don their PPE?
- What will staff wear under their PPE, including footwear?
- Can staff don and doff independently or will they need assistance?
- Is there a chair, stepstool, or grab bar available where donning and doffing occur?
- How long will each professional likely remain in the room delivering care?
- Will the staff sanitize their PPE in some manner before or during doffing?
- Where will staff doff?
- Is there a mirror for staff to check their PPE?
- Can staff be observed while doffing?
- Will you use a trained observer?
  - What will a trained observer wear?
  - What PPE will ancillary personnel, such as environmental services, wear?
- If PPE is reusable, who cleans it and what is worn while it is being cleaned?

Putting together the best PPE ensemble depends on availability, price, ease of use, and the amount and type of protection required. In the USA, most of the gowns and suits worn for isolation purposes are disposable, contrary to the reusable suits

Table 14.2 Fabric standards for protective clothing [12]

National standards and what they mean for PPE			
ANSI/AAMI standards			
Level	Test methods	Barrier effect	Limitations
1	Impact penetration (water splash)	Minimal – Some resistance to water spray	Only tested on water which has a higher surface tension than many body fluids
2	Impact penetration with hydrostatic pressure	Low – Resistance to spray and some resistance to water penetration under pressure	
3	Impact penetration and increasing hydrostatic pressure	Moderate – Resistance to water spray and some resistance to water penetration with constant contact or increasing pressure	
4	ASTM F1670 synthetic blood and ASTM F1671 viral penetration	Blood and viral penetration resistance	

worn in most of Europe [11]. It is imperative that infection prevention personnel, supervisors, and purchasing agents all understand what items are being used in the biocontainment unit or with the care of any patient with a highly hazardous communicable disease and what level of protection they provide. International standards exist for the fabrics gowns are made from, as shown in Table 14.2.

It is important for those planning, purchasing, and writing protocols for the use of PPE suits and gowns to recognize that only Level 4 material has been tested using fluids with lower specific gravity than water, which is true of most bodily fluids [12]. Materials in Levels 1–3 have not been tested with fluids of similar specific gravity to bile, blood, or liquid stool and may have no resistance to these.

Choosing PPE that provides the highest level of protection against synthetic blood and simulated blood-borne pathogens exclusively allows staff to train in and use one ensemble that provides protection against various pathogens regardless of their transmission route. While it may be argued that this is "over-isolating," this approach mitigates concerns when dealing with new pathogens, unknown pathogens, or as information emerges about the existence and persistence of pathogens in varying body fluids [8].

Risks to PPE exist in varying forms. Defects in manufacturing and assembly can leave seams and zippers open to penetration. Both the person donning and the trained observer should inspect PPE as it is being put on. Suit materials can be torn or cut by sharp edges within the environment, and breaches in suit integrity can occur with use while staff bend, stoop, and reach. Special populations of patients can also pose hazards to PPE integrity by grabbing, pulling, or holding onto staff. Whether intentional or unintentional, the potential for a contaminating breach must be mitigated by the care team to the extent it is possible and foreseeable. Patients, who are delirious or agitated, frightened, or simply active as in the case of toddlers, pose higher risks to staff and to the integrity of a PPE ensemble. If a breach occurs, protocols must be in place first to guide the staff member in the safest extrication from danger and then to assess, treat, and monitor the employee as needed.

Gowns and Suits

Gown and suit choice should consider ease of donning and doffing, as well as how it functions during use. Gowns are generally easier and safer for staff to don, may be more familiar to HCW, and usually can be put on without assistance. Some other considerations for gowns involve a fit that does not allow the front of the gown to touch the floor when performing patient care tasks, that covers the entire back of the wearer, and that remains securely positioned during use.

Suit style PPE can offer additional coverage of underclothing, does not have a risk of falling off shoulders in use, and does not drape the floor with bending or stooping, but is more difficult to don and, because of sizing limitations, may fit better in certain areas of the body than others. Employees should know which size of suit fits them safely, reducing redundant fabric without compromising the wearer's ability to bend, crouch, or sit. Seams and zippers, if any, should be covered. Donning and doffing suit style PPE is a skill that should be practiced and considered a part of staff competency.

Both gown and suit style PPE compliant with the Level 4 ASTM/AMSI standards are fluid impervious under pressure, which is beneficial for many of the intimate contact tasks that may be required while caring for patients. An unintended consequence of that fluid repellence is an increased risk of liquid and body fluid running off to the lower legs, shoes, and floor. Boot and shoe covers should be worn [13]. If gowns are used, shoe covers should extend to an area higher on the leg than the lowest portion of the gown. Suits with built-in "booties" should be worn with shoe covers that can be changed in the case of gross contamination (Figs. 14.1 and 14.2).

Gloves

Gloves and glove etiquette is another area where familiarity with a product does not necessarily infer safe use. Staff may need to practice methods of glove removal that discourage contamination, whether a glove-in-glove or other method is utilized. Fluorescing solutions and UV flashlights make this an easy exercise and one that is key to good technique. Studies have demonstrated an increased safety to staff with double gloving, but most of these determinations were made when the threat to the staff was from substances such as bone cements and glues [2]. Double gloving by itself does not prevent contamination of the wearer from either poor technique or from unrecognized loss of glove integrity [14]. Balancing the need for increased protection with required tactile sensation is not easy. Staff will need practice performing required skills while in extra layers of gloves. Because the cuffs of gowns and suits are not required to be fluid impervious, it is important that gloves extend over that portion completely and may require the use of an extended cuff glove [11].

Fig. 14.1 Emory PPE

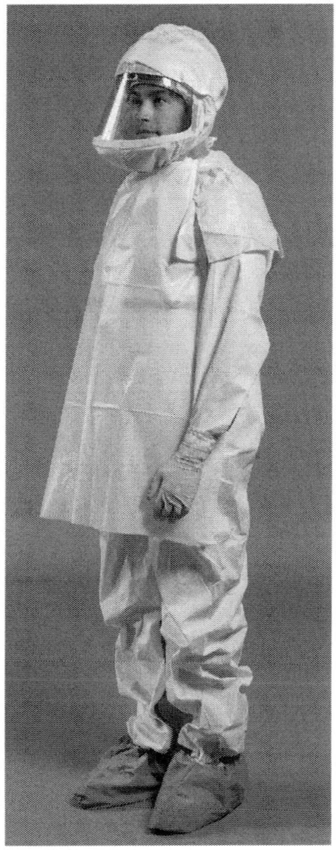

Some institutions have chosen to use longer and heartier sterile gloves as their outer layer, while others have opted for extended cuff length exam gloves designed for chemotherapy use to offer a similar level of protection. Triple gloving is another option, which provides an additional glove which can be exchanged during patient care activities.

The use of alcohol-based hand rubs (ABHRs) on gloved hands allows for sanitizing without exposing skin while in a patient care area. The application of alcohol-based hand rubs has not been shown to have a negative effect on the gloves themselves [15], at least during limited use. Sanitizing the outer layer of gloves after touching the patient or a patient care device or surface is an important step in reducing further contamination of the care space. When outer gloves have been in contact with known areas of contamination or with patient body fluids, they should be sanitized and then changed [2].

Another strategy for glove safety is to employ gloves that are different in color layer to layer. This allows a visual queue when the outer glove has been compromised. Gloves should be inspected when they are donned and again before they are doffed to ensure that they have remained intact. Breaches in glove integrity, if they

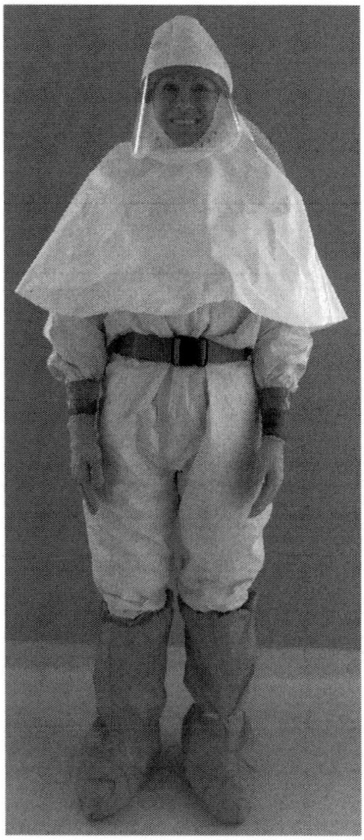

Fig. 14.2 Nebraska Biocontainment Unit PAPR level PPE

involve both layers or the inner layer alone, should be regarded as a potential staff exposure.

To provide a continuous impervious surface along the hand, wrist, and forearm, some facilities tape their gloves to their suits or gowns. Decisions to tape gloves should be considered in the larger context of the donning and doffing procedure to ensure that staff understand both the rational and the timing of applying and removing tape. The benefit of a smooth, continuous wipeable surface in one of the high-risk zones for contamination must be weighed against the risk for damage to the suit or gown, the potential of micro-spray created during tape removal, and adding complexity to the donning and doffing procedure.

Droplet- and aerosol-generating procedures and situations can be abrupt and unpredictable. They include coughing without appropriate mouth coverage; sneezing; spitting; suctioning; pouring liquid waste into toilet; emptying bedpans, catheter bags, or urinals; and being near patients when they are urinating or defecating, or when staff assist with activities such as tooth brushing. A powered air-purifying respirator provides the greatest and most complete protection from these potential events, especially for caregivers within the critical 3-foot zone around the patient [16]. For facilities and staff who do not have access to or have not been trained in the use of these respirators, an N95 face mask and shield or a N95 face mask and goggles may need to be used.

Face Shields/Goggles

While likely less protective than the enclosed head piece of a powered air-purifying respirator (PAPR), for short periods of time in biocontainment units, or when patients are no longer exhibiting symptoms, a combination of face shield or goggles and a mask may be used. Eye protection serves to avoid the two mechanisms for worker exposure – direct splash into the eyes and self-inoculation with contaminated hands. Goggles, like eyeglasses, may move on the face during wear, tempting the wearer to reach up and adjust them with contaminated hands. Face shields have the advantage of being able to be worn with eyeglasses. Top-down full face shields lend more protection as users lean forward while delivering care than the smaller shields that are attached to surgical type masks, which can expose eyes to sprays and droplets when the wearers head is down.

Masks

Masks fall into two larger categories, isolation type single use and the N95 respirator [17]. An N95 or its equivalent in protection, or a PAPR, is required for all airborne pathogens as well as high-consequence pathogens when the care of the patient requires staff members to be within 3 feet of the patient's mouth and nose and when that patient is coughing and sneezing or has copious oral or nasal secretions. Again, because aerosol-generating incidents, such as a sneeze, can occur without warning, when staff are required to be in very proximity to any patient suffering from high-consequence pathogens, appropriate eye, nose, and mouth coverage should be maintained. An isolation type surgical mask may be worn in conjunction with a face shield to prevent the direct inoculation of staff mucous membranes only when there is not a risk of airborne transmission.

Mask removal must occur with clean hands, and staff should be encouraged not to touch their faces, eyes, nose, or mouth until they have thoroughly washed. Once a mask has been used, it should be discarded.

Powered Air-Purifying Respirators

As is true with other types of personal protective equipment, PAPRs require training and practice to be used effectively and efficiently. With highly hazardous communicable diseases, ease of use is a lesser factor than the protection that a piece of equipment provides. Surgical masks are the easiest for wearers to put on and take off correctly. N95 masks require training and fitting and annual competency [18]. PAPRs require training and practice, and many facilities using PAPRs have staff retrain on a more frequent basis.

Generally, the PAPR motor and fan are attached to or contiguous with head covering that contains a large face shield. Airflow is directed past the face to maintain a continuous positive pressure inside the face portion of the hood. Motors, and the

Table 14.3 Pros and cons of powered air-purifying respirators

Advantages	Disadvantages
Comfort	Expensive
Increased wear time	Require practice and training
Good visibility	Require power source
Stability with movement	Produce noise and impair hearing
Increased protection from N95	External hose, when present, risk entanglement
Full face, hair, head, and neck coverage	Not all hoods or portions of hoods are impervious
Less risk of fogging	

battery pack powering them, can either be worn on a belt at the waist or can be integral to the helmet structure beneath a disposable hood. Care must be taken to assure that a battery pack does not lose power while in use.

PAPRs may offer improvement in comfort and cooling compared to N95 masks and face shields or goggles. When workers wear PPE longer and more comfortably, they can stay at the bedside longer, reducing the number of required doffings per day. This can substantially reduce overall risk as each doffing episode confers risk of contamination to staff and the work environment [14] (Table 14.3).

Other PPE

Additions to the PPE ensemble may be aprons, gowns, shoe covers, and hair/head covers. Hats and hair covers may be integral to the hood or head piece or may be applied separately. Generally, these hair covers must also be impervious if they serve as the outermost layer. Care should be taken to ensure that they do not slip or move while being worn and do not compromise visibility.

Aprons and gowns can help create a smooth wipeable surface on the front high-risk area of the wearer, mitigating the risk along seam and zipper lines. Aprons afford covering to the chest and torso, while surgical or plastic gowns add protection to the arms. Each addition to the PPE ensemble must also be considered with relation to where the item will fit in the donning and doffing procedures. Staff should consider whether these items can be safely cleaned while in use, with sanitizing wipes, or whether they can be removed and replaced safely while within the patient care environment. The addition of a gown or apron is now recommended by the CDC as the outermost layer of a PPE ensemble as it avoids the folds and seams of underlying fabrics and can provide a wipeable surface and allows for additional protection in what are considered the high-touch areas of the anterior chest, torso, and arms [12].

Shoe covers are utilized over existing foot and lower leg coverage to allow the outer layer to be removed if soiled. Soiling of the shoe and lower leg areas can occur from splashes of body fluids that fall from the impervious layers of the PPE above them as well as from spills and splashes that reach the floor. Protocols for staff are needed to ensure that they can remove and replace contaminated foot coverings if needed, especially during the cleanup of spills. Suits that have built-in foot coverings should still have a removable foot covering added for likely contamination events.

Trained Observer

The duty of a trained observer in a biocontainment unit is like that of a safety officer, watching but not participating in patient care, donning and doffing, unless needed in an emergency. In such a case, another trained individual should be ready and able to step in to the role of trained observer. The role is not designed as punitive or for score keeping but for identifying potential breaches that could compromise safety. It is not possible for staff in full PPE to know when a portion of their ensemble has come in contact with the patient or part of the environment. Even with practice, bedside caregivers may occasionally omit hand hygiene or a step in the doffing process. All members of the care team should be aware of the actions of those around them and be watchful for omissions that could compromise safety.

PPE Etiquette

By itself, no PPE ensemble protects staff if it is not used and maintained properly. PPE etiquette involves every step a staff member takes while providing safe patient care, from avoiding touching their own PPE and hand hygiene while gloved, to proper cleaning of PAPR motors, helmets, and belts. Gloved hands can be sanitized with alcohol-based hand rubs (ABHRs) but should not be washed while in the patient care environment to avoid splashing. Beds and bed linens, doors, tables and chairs, and all items within easy reach of the patient, such as TV remotes and call lights should be considered contaminated even without visible soiling. Once a staff member has touched those high-risk areas, they should perform hand hygiene or change outer gloves. Cleaning those areas of high risk repeatedly becomes part of the work day for clinicians at the bedside of the patient with a highly hazardous communicable disease.

Performing tasks that are normally routine for staff can pose hazards when performed in PPE, so they should be practiced and drilled. Staff proprioception is altered in their PPE, and developing a new sense of where the edges of their PPE-encapsulated body are in space is vital. Through practice, staff can become accustomed to the hoses, battery packs, helmets, hoods, and boot covers that alter this proprioception.

Mindfulness of where and what has been touched during the performance of clinical duties can be augmented by using a trained observer but is ultimately a change in the fundamental way staff deliver care. Clinicians must become keen observers of what surfaces and objects a patient may have contacted, from call lights and bedside tables to door handles, bed rails, and bathroom fixtures. Every action inside the patient care area must be taken with safety in mind, avoiding those hazards that can be difficult to see while in a PAPR or face shield, to feel while double gloved, or to hear due to the background hum of the PAPR motor.

Doffing

As employees prepare to leave the patient care area, they should examine their PPE for breaches and visible soiling. Sanitizing wipes may be used to clean high-risk or likely soiled areas of PPE. A trained observer may be used outside the patient room, or in an anteroom or hallway, to observe the doffing process. If the observing staff is not separated by a physical barrier such as a wall, door, or window, they must be protected from potential splashes that can occur during the removal of PPE or be in PPE themselves.

A mirror may be helpful for the staff member to see their entire ensemble. The doffing protocol may be posted so that both the person doffing and their trained partner can ensure that each step is followed, or staff can follow an electronic version that records their compliance.

Each PPE ensemble will require a unique doffing protocol and many employ the use of ABHRs or other sanitizing devices such as UV light sources to reduce the risk of contamination during the doffing process [19]. A step-by-step approach avoids errors that can result in the unapparent transfer of infective materials. Where doffing occurs will be best determined by the physical layout of the unit and the space available but should occur a minimum of 6 feet from the patient in an area that has been dedicated to this purpose and is maintained as cleanly as possible.

Once the entire PPE ensemble has been doffed and the staff member is outside of the direct patient care area, they should be reminded not to touch any part of their bodies until they have thoroughly washed their hands. This final redundancy prevents indirect inoculation of staff from disposing of their used PPE.

Conclusion

Perhaps one of the greatest challenges when clinical duties require PPE is for HCWs to place the safety of themselves and their team first. Nothing, including the sudden loss of airway patency, consciousness, or pulse, should drive a clinician into the room of a patient with a highly hazardous communicable disease without proper PPE. Being mindful of how long it can take to don PPE and how difficult it can be to move both quickly and safely in the patient environment means that staff members in biocontainment units must be even more vigilant than usual in observing patients for early signs of decline in condition. The ability to anticipate critical needs can prevent staff from reacting dangerously and without the proper PPE. We must consider the patient care area to be our scene, and our first question must remain, is the scene safe? The right PPE, donned in the correct order, worn in a safe manner, is what makes that scene safe for bedside healthcare providers. The safe, observed, step-by-step doffing of PPE is what ensures the safety of the rest of the unit, staff, and facility.

While healthcare workers use PPE routinely, we are also responsible for at least some of the nosocomial infections that plague modern healthcare facilities. In bio-containment units, as well as many other areas in the healthcare system, such microbe spread can have deadly consequences. Research is needed to determine best practice with respect to PPE, including the type of gloves and glove removal techniques that avoid hand and clothing contamination. Development of PPE suits that fit all sizes and meet the needs of the bedside clinician is also necessary. Decontamination procedures for reusable suits that are efficacious and cost-effective could reduce the enormous cost associated with the disposable suits now in use.

In addition, behavioral research could lend credence to the frequency, timing, and scope of PPE training and protocols for doffing that are proven to reduce staff contamination. New technologies in sanitation, including the use of ultraviolet light, may reduce in-room fomites. The future is likely to be filled with larger and more frequent outbreaks of highly hazardous communicable diseases. When we can be assured that HCWs are using the right PPE with good PPE etiquette and following protocols that have been validated through robust research, the healthcare setting will be safer for everyone.

References

1. Garner, JS, Simmons BP. Guideline for isolation precautions in hospitals. [Online]. 1996 [cited 2016 Dec 27]; CDC Prevention Guidelines Database (Archive). Available from: URL:https://wonder.cdc.gov/wonder/prevguid/p0000419/p0000419.asp#head002003000000000.
2. Graves PB, Twomey CL. The changing face of hand protection. AORN J [Online from PubMed] 2002 Aug [2016 Dec 27]; 76(2):246–58.
3. Nutton V. The reception of Fracastoro's theory of contagion: the seed that fell among thorns? [Online from The University of Chicago Press Journals]. 1990 [2016 Dec 27]; 6i:196–234. Available from: URL:www.journals.uchicago.edu/doi/abs/10.1086/368701.
4. Grady D. Questions rise on preparedness at hospitals to deal with Ebola. (Internet) New York Times. 2014 Oct 13 [cited 2016 Dec 29]; Available from: https://www.nytimes/2014/10/14/US/questions-rise-on-preparations-at-hospitals-to-deal-with-ebola.html.
5. Fuller TP. Personal protective equipment: patient and worker safety. In: Charney W, editor. Epidemic of medical errors and hospital-acquired infections: systemic and social causes [Internet]. Boca Raton: CRC Press; 2012 [cited 2016 Dec 29].
6. Casanova L, Alfano-Sobsey E, Rutala WA, Weber DJ, Sobsey M. Virus transfer from personal protective equipment to healthcare employees' skin and clothing. Emerg Infect Dis 2008;14(8):1291–3. Available from: https://doi.org/10.3201/eid1408.080085.
7. Casanova LM, Rutala WA, Weber DJ, Sobsey MD. Effect of single-versus double-gloving on virus transfer to health care workers' skin and clothing during removal of personal protective equipment. Am J Infect Control [Internet]. 2012 [cited 2016 Dec 29]; 40(4):369–74. Available from: PubMed.
8. US Department of Health, Education, and welfare. Isolation techniques for use in hospitals. Washington, DC: Public Health Service Publication 2054; US Government Printing Office; 1970.
9. CDC. Guidance on personal protective equipment (PPE) to be used by healthcare workers during management of patients with confirmed Ebola or persons under investigation (PUI's)

for Ebola who are clinically unstable or have bleeding, vomiting, or diarrhea in US hospitals, including procedures for donning and doffing PPE. [Online] 2015 Aug 27 [cited 2016 Dec 29]. Available from: https://www.cdc.gov/vhf/ebola/healthcare-us/ppe/guidance.html.

10. Larson EL, Liverman CT, Institute of Medicine (US) Committee on Personal Protective Equipment. Preventing transmission of pandemic influenza and other respiratory diseases [Internet]. Washington, DC: National Academies Press; 2014 [cited 2016 Dec 29]. Available from: PubMed.
11. Kilinc FS. A review of isolation gowns in healthcare: fabric and gown properties. J Eng Fiber Fabr. 2015 Jul [cited 2016 Dec 29]; 10(3):180–90. Available from: PubMed.
12. CDC. Considerations for selecting protective clothing used in healthcare for protection against microorganisms in blood and body fluids. 2015 Feb 10. [cited 2016 Dec 29]. Available from: https://www.cdc.gov/niosh/npptl/topics/protectiveclothing/default.html.
13. Guo YP, Li Y, Wong PL. Environment and body contamination: a comparison of two different removal methods in three types of personal protective clothing. Am J Infect Control [Internet]. 2014 Apr [cited 2016 Dec 26];42(4):39–45. Available from: PubMed.
14. Casanova LM, Teal LJ, Sickbert-Bennett EE, Anderson DJ, Sexton DJ, Rutala WA, et al. Assessment of self-contamination during removal of personal protective equipment for Ebola patient care. Infect Control Hosp Epidemiol [Internet]. 2016 Oct [cited 2016 Dec 29];37(10):1156–61. Available from: PubMed.
15. Gao P, Horvatin M, Niezgoda G, Weible R, Shaffer R. Effect of multiple alcohol-based hand rub applications on the tensile properties of thirteen brands of medical exam nitrile and latex gloves. J Occup Environ Hyg [Internet]. 2016 Dec [cited 2016 Dec 29];13(12):905–14. Available from: PubMed.
16. Siegel JD, Rhinehart E, Jackson M, Chiarello L, Health Care Infection Control Practices Advisory Committee. 2007 Guideline for isolation precautions: preventing transmission of infectious agents in health care settings. Am J Infect Control [Internet]. 2007 Dec [cited 2016 Dec 29];35(10) Suppl 2:s65–164, Available from: https://doi.org/10.1016/j.ajic.2007.10.007.
17. National Personal Protective Technology Laboratory. NIOSH- Approved N95 particulate filtering facepiece respirators. [Internet]. Updated 2014 Sep [cited 2016 Dec 27]. Available from: https://www.cdc.gov/niosh/npptl/topics/respirators/disp_part/h95list1.html.
18. United States Department of Labor. Personal protective equipment standard # 1910.134 App. A. [Internet]. Occupational Safety and Health Administration Occupational Safety and Health Standards. [cited 2016 Dec 29]. Available from: https://www.osha.gov/pls/oshaweb/owadisp.show_document?p_table=standards&p_id=9780.
19. Jinadatha C, Simmons S, Dale C, Ganachari-Mallapa N, Villamaria FC, Goulding N, Tanner B, et al. Disinfecting personal protective equipment with pulsed xenon ultraviolet as a risk mitigation strategy for health care workers. Am J Infect Control [Internet]. 2015 Apr [cited 2016 Dec 27];43(4):412–4. Available from: PubMed.

Human Subjects Research in Bioemergencies

15

Lauren M. Sauer, Jared D. Evans, Kathryn Shaw-Saliba, Bruce Gordon, and Christopher J. Kratochvil

Introduction

The nature of clinical care in bioemergencies presents distinct ethical and operational challenges for both patient care and research. While the most pressing concern at the onset of a bioemergency is always implementing clinical and public health measures to mitigate impact and stop the spread of disease, research is still needed to support this goal and improve our capacity to respond to the next threat.

As research within the context of containment care (i.e., patient care within a clinical biocontainment unit) remains a relatively new domain, novel and unexpected challenges present themselves as research opportunities that are approached in each new bioemergency. These challenges will vary greatly depending on the type of research being conducted. Understanding basic broad principles of the human subjects research relevant to studies conducted in acute care settings, as well as the growing experiences of investigators in these unique settings, will develop an informed foundation for containment care investigators.

L. M. Sauer (✉)
Johns Hopkins Biocontainment Unit, Johns Hopkins Hospital, Baltimore, MD, USA

Department of Emergency Medicine, Johns Hopkins University, Baltimore, MD, USA
e-mail: lsauer2@jhmi.edu

J. D. Evans
Department of Emergency Medicine, Johns Hopkins University, Baltimore, MD, USA

Research and Exploratory Development Department, Johns Hopkins University Applied Physics Laboratory, Laurel, MD, USA

K. Shaw-Saliba
Department of Emergency Medicine, Johns Hopkins University School of Medicine, Baltimore, MD, USA

B. Gordon · C. J. Kratochvil
University of Nebraska Medical Center, Omaha, NE, USA

A. Hewlett, A. R. K. Murthy (eds.), *Bioemergency Planning*,
https://doi.org/10.1007/978-3-319-77032-1_15

Recent pandemic threats (severe acute respiratory syndrome (SARS), avian influenza H5N1, pandemic influenza H1N1, and the 2014 Ebola virus disease outbreak) have highlighted the challenges in conducting clinical research in disease outbreaks, particularly involving novel or (re)emerging pathogens, particularly those about which limited systematic or high-quality data are available. Moreover, a debate has arisen regarding the ethical basis of the clinical and public health research being conducted during these emergencies. Research opportunities in bioemergencies are ample, and a number of considerations must be taken into account to ensure patient, public, and care worker safety. Conducting effective research in these environments requires making the distinction between it and public health practice or operational response [1].

Research Opportunities in Clinical Biocontainment Units

Clinical biocontainment units provide a novel but challenging platform for research in bioemergencies. Despite the broadly recognized importance of this research, international and domestic ethics guiding principles, as well as basic human rights, must be upheld and protected. Critical to these efforts is distinguishing the difference between data collection and analysis for effective response and clinical practice in an operational response and human subjects research for generalizable knowledge. To make this distinction, one must address the intent of the activity, which easily becomes blurred during emergencies [1]. For example, in a recent outbreak of Middle East respiratory syndrome coronavirus (MERS Co-V), epidemiologic and clinical data were collected and analyzed to determine the most effective infection control measures. The goal of this investigation was to effectively reduce transmission of MERS Co-V; however, the data will ultimately inform broader research questions outside of the context of the outbreak.

A critical priority for clinical and public health researchers, particularly those who are also practitioners, is understanding how to determine what activities are human subjects research versus a "standard" clinical operational response. To answer this question, the investigator must determine his or her goal. The Health and Human Services Office for Human Research Protections provides guidance on whether an activity is human subjects research [2]. Figure 15.1 demonstrates a decision tree for determining whether or not an individual is performing human subjects research. If the goal of the investigation is to develop or contribute to generalizable knowledge, this is fundamentally research and must progress down the regulatory path associated with research.

Research Types

There are several research activities that can be conducted in bioemergencies. In this chapter, we will focus primarily on clinical research, particularly as it relates to human subjects participation in bioemergencies. Among the various types of

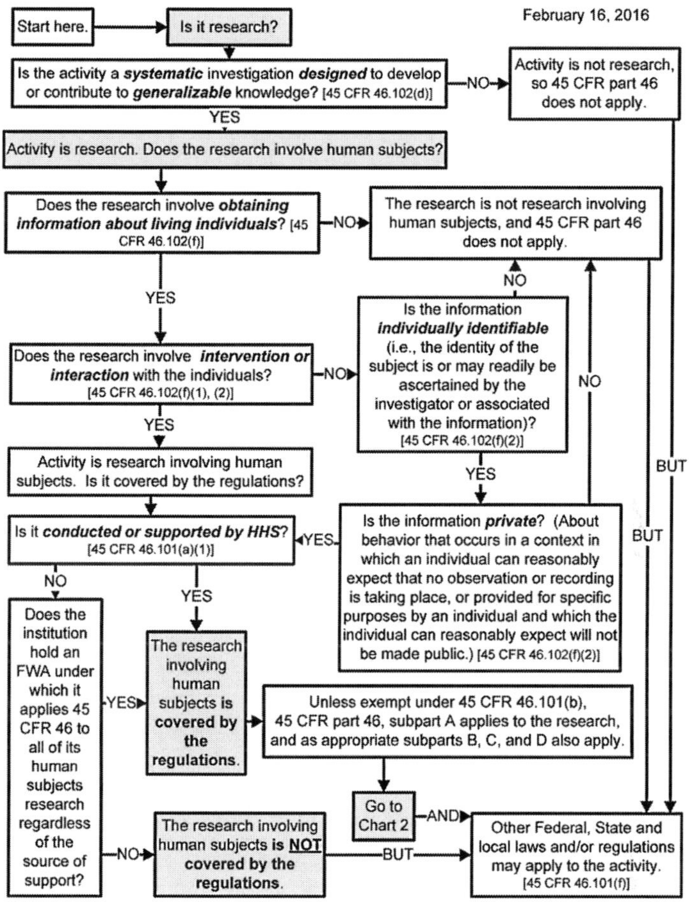

Fig. 15.1 Decision chart to determine if an activity is research involving human subjects. (From: Human Subject Regulations Decision Charts [Internet]. HHS.gov. 2016 [cited 26 October 2017]. Available from: https://www.hhs.gov/ohrp/regulations-and-policy/decision-charts/index.html#c1)

clinical research, treatment studies are the most likely, as they generally involve analyzing the effects of a countermeasure, therapeutic, or other intervention on affected or at-risk individuals.

Additionally, research related to vaccine or postexposure prophylaxis development and trials in an at-risk population, such as healthcare workers, may be conducted, with the goal of developing therapeutics and other tools for prevention of future outbreaks/infections. Other examples of research may involve collection of biospecimens for use in future research efforts or quarantine or containment research to understand infection and transmission dynamics. Research specimens are highly valuable in informing downstream laboratory analysis for better understanding of infectious diseases. Finally, diagnostic and screening research seeks to detect specific diseases or individuals afflicted by them. These studies offer new information on a critical component of research in outbreaks and pandemics, as it focuses on preventing further spread of the infection.

Other research is necessary for an effective clinical and public health response beyond clinical research. Operational or implementation research in bioemergencies often focuses on real-time improvements to the clinical or health system response. This may include epidemiological studies focused on identification of causes, effects, or simply cases of a specific infection and may include looking for patterns during an outbreak for improved response, and many of these cases may not constitute human subjects research.

Regulatory Oversight of Human Subjects Research in Bioemergencies

The basic protections for human subjects of research are promulgated in the Common Rule, published in 1991, and based on the HHS regulations at 45 Code of Federal Regulations [CFR] part 46 [3]. The Common Rule applies to research conducted or supported by any of the departments and agencies that are signatories to the rule. Additional regulations at 21 CFR 50 (Protection of Human Subjects) and 21 CFR 56 (IRBs) cover clinical investigations using FDA-regulated products and differ only slightly from the HHS regulations.

These rules generally lay out the specific requirements for Institutional Review Board (IRB) operations and the conditions under which human subjects research may occur. This includes, among other things, the specific criteria for approval of research by the IRB, the process of obtaining informed consent from human subjects, and the elements of information that must be part of that process.

The IRB must assure that certain conditions are met before approving human subjects research. These criteria for approval are based on the ethical principles of respect for persons, beneficence, and justice, as laid out in the Belmont Report [3]. The IRB must judge that risks to subjects are minimized, that the risks are reasonable in relation to anticipated benefits to subject or to society, that subject selection is equitable, that informed consent is obtained, and that additional safeguards have been included to protect the vulnerable subjects, as well as other requirements.

Research conducted in the setting of a bioemergency presents challenges to both the investigator and to the IRB in assuring that these ethical and regulatory requirements are met so that critical research can be conducted.

Risk/Benefit

Research must be conducted in a manner that minimizes risk to participants. The investigator must design the protocol to limit potential harms, must monitor subjects throughout the protocol, and be prepared to adjust study parameters or design to assure that the subjects are not exposed to unnecessary risk. At the same time the protocol must be designed to maximize the possibility of direct subject benefit and of more general scientific value. This may be particularly difficult in the setting of a disease process with an unknown natural history while using interventions of unproven (and, in many cases, only theoretical) efficacy.

Subject Selection

In all research, the ethical principles of the Belmont Report and HHS and FDA regulations require that selection of subjects must be fair and primarily based on scientific validity but also distribute risks and benefits equitably. This is particularly true in the case of therapeutic research during bioemergencies.

Where availability of interventions is limited, priorities should be dictated by ethical principles such as fairness between countries and among populations within countries (i.e., distributive justice) and the likelihood of a positive impact on both individual and public health outcomes. In addition, investigators should consider issues of reciprocity and social usefulness. Reciprocity refers to the obligations of healthcare workers during a pandemic and the obligations of society to them in return; that is, the acceptance of a healthcare provider's risk taking care of a patient with a highly communicable disease engenders reciprocal duties on the part of the community to them. Social usefulness refers to the idea that healthcare workers preferential access to prophylaxis and treatment would be directly associated with the continued ability of the healthcare system to provide interventions to everybody else [4].

Informed Consent

The investigator must design the study, and the IRB must also be assured that subjects will provide their voluntary and valid informed consent before participating in the research and that such consent is based on adequate, understandable information presented in a manner that minimizes the possibility of confusion, coercion, or undue influence. The conditions surrounding a bioemergency do not easily lend themselves to the provision of time for thoughtful consideration by a subject nor can the investigator be sure of the risks associated with his or her interventions, much less clearly explain them to a subject.

Further, subjects may be too ill to meaningfully or practically participate in the process of informed consent (particularly with some of the special pathogens such as Ebola virus that can contribute to substantial cognitive impairment). Under these circumstances, it may be necessary to utilize a legally authorized representative to provide "consent" (more accurately, "permission") for the patient to participate in the research.

Waiver of consent for participation in research is allowed under FDA and HHS regulations in very limited circumstances. FDA regulations allow that informed consent may be waived if the investigator and a physician who is not otherwise participating in the clinical investigation certify in writing that (1) the human subject is confronted by a life-threatening situation necessitating the use of the test article; (2) informed consent cannot be obtained from the subject because of an inability to communicate with, or obtain legally effective consent from, the subject; (3) time is not sufficient to obtain consent from the subject's legal representative; and (4) there is no available alternative method of approved or generally recognized therapy that provides an equal or greater likelihood of saving the life of the subject [5]. While potentially applicable to treatment studies of novel interventions for incapacitated persons in a bioemergency, such waiver would not be appropriate for collection of biospecimens or epidemiologic studies.

In addition FDA allows for exception from informed consent requirements for emergency research [6]; however, conducting research under these regulations requires extensive preparation and investigator and IRB responsibilities. For example, the regulations require consultation with representatives of and public disclosure to the communities in which the clinical investigation will be conducted and from which the subjects will be drawn, prior to initiation of the clinical investigation. They also require public disclosure of sufficient information following completion of the clinical investigation to apprise the community and researchers of the study. As well, the regulations require that an independent data monitoring committee exercises oversight of the clinical investigation. These additional protections make use of this method unsuitable for most bioemergency situations.

It is important to stress that consent to participate in therapy research during a bioemergency is different from consent in the clinical treatment setting. In the clinical setting, for patients who are incapacitated, in need of a lifesaving intervention, and who cannot provide consent, "implied consent" is acceptable practice. "Implied consent" is not valid in the research setting.

Additional FDA Considerations

Under FDA regulations, the use of an FDA-unapproved drug, device, or biologic on a human subject requires, except under very limited circumstances, prior IRB approval. The use also requires informed consent (except as described above).

The usual process requires that the FDA grants an investigational new drug (IND), or an investigational device exemption (IDE) designation, which allows the drug or device to be used before it is legally marketed. Considering the use of unapproved drugs, most commonly, an investigator or a sponsor submits an IND to propose studying an unapproved drug or an approved product for a new indication or in a new patient population. In contrast, an emergency use IND allows the FDA to authorize use of an experimental drug in an emergency situation that does not allow time for the usual IND process. It is also used for patients who do not meet the criteria of an existing study protocol or if an approved study protocol does not exist. Finally, a treatment IND may be submitted for experimental drugs showing promise in clinical testing for serious or immediately life-threatening conditions while the final clinical work is conducted and the FDA review takes place [7].

Research utilizing drugs under any of these three types of INDs requires IRB approval. As described above, the IRB must determine that the criteria for approval are met, that informed consent is obtained, and that the rights and welfare of the subject are protected.

Under very specific and limited circumstances, unapproved drugs may be used without prospective IRB approval. FDA regulations allow for use of an investigational drug or biological product in a life-threatening situation in which no standard acceptable treatment is available and in which there is not sufficient time to obtain IRB approval [8]. The regulation allows for one emergency use of a test article without prospective IRB review; subsequent use of the investigational product at the institution has prospective IRB review and approval. FDA acknowledges, however, that it would be inappropriate to deny emergency treatment to a ond individual if the only obstacle is that the IRB has not had sufficient time to convene a meeting to review the issue. Even for an emergency use, the investigator is required to obtain informed consent of the subject or the subject's legally authorized representative (except as has been described above).

A second mechanism for use of unapproved drugs in a bioemergency involves the issuance of an emergency use authorization (EUA) [9]. The FDA may allow unapproved medical products or unapproved uses of approved medical products to be used in an emergency to diagnose, treat, or prevent serious or life-threatening diseases or conditions caused by biological agents (like Ebola or anthrax) when there are no adequate, approved, and available alternatives. The EUA must be issued by the commissioner based on a determination by the secretary of Homeland Security, Defense, or HHS, that a domestic, military, or public health emergency exists. Products approved under an EUA must meet a (lower) standard of effectiveness, must address a serious or life-threatening disease or condition, must have a favorable risk-benefit assessment, and must have no adequate, approved, and available alternative. The EUA is valid for up to 1 year from the date of the declaration of emergency or for as long as the emergency is in effect, whichever is shorter.

Use of a drug or device under an EUA requires neither IRB review nor informed consent (though a "fact sheet" for healthcare providers and recipients is required).

IRB Review

As discussed above, IRBs are responsible for protecting the rights and welfare of human subjects of research, a responsivity shared, obviously, with the investigator. The IRB must determine that the regulatory criteria for approval are met. Typically, the IRB receives a written application describing the research, as well as the investigators description of how the investigator will assure that risks are minimized, the risk benefit relationship is acceptable, subject selection is equitable, and so on. The IRB reviews this information (along with the full sponsor protocol, the informed consent documents, the investigator's brochure, and any additional materials) at a full convened meeting. After due deliberation, the board may approve the research conditional upon minor modifications or return the application to the investigator for clarification or modifications needed to satisfy the regulatory criteria for approval. In addition, review and approval by other committees (scientific review, Pharmacy and Therapeutics, Sponsored Programs and Contracts, Institutional Biosafety) may be needed. Eventually, the protocol is approved, and the investigator may begin recruiting potential subjects. The process is thoughtful and protective but does not typically lend itself to the urgent timeline associated with a bioemergency.

Several approaches to this problem have been utilized. For example, the Ethics Review Board for Médecins Sans Frontières (MSF) has described a process of review and approval of a generic pathogen or intervention agnostic master research protocol in advance of a bioemergency; the details related to the specifics of the outbreak are then amended to the protocol when known [10].

Another approach has been the creation of national or regional central IRBs, with focus on public health emergencies, including bioemergencies. The HHS Public Health Emergency Research Review Board (PHERRB) is one such body and can serve as the IRB of record for any institution (such as a state health department, academic medical center, or community hospital) that is engaged in the conduct of the protocol [11].

A third approach is the utilization of a "Rapid Response IRB" such as that developed at the University of Nebraska Medical Center (UNMC). This fully constituted IRB was created to allow for review of clinical protocols on an expedited timeline, utilizing extensive prereview of protocols and consent documents in an iterative process, and close collaboration with the investigator. The UNMC Rapid Response IRB (RR-IRB) was used successfully to review research protocols associated with several investigational drugs and interventions targeting patients with Ebola virus disease hospitalized in the Nebraska Biocontainment Unit at UNMC/Nebraska Medicine.

The RR-IRB at UNMC also serves as the central IRB for the entire National Ebola Training and Education Center (NETEC) Special Pathogens Research Network, consisting of UNMC and the nine additional NETEC regional treatment center sites [12]. To facilitate this single IRB process, the network utilizes the reliance agreements modeled by the NIH SMART (Streamlined, Multisite, Accelerated Resources for Trials) IRB Platform [13].

Practical Issues

One of the biggest challenges of conducting research in bioemergencies is that they often involve novel disease-causing agents or pathogens. When the pathogen is novel, predetermined study design and pre-identification of affected populations and countermeasures is almost impossible [14]. This challenge represents situations where research, particularly clinical studies, is most needed as novel diseases often do not have associated therapeutics that are far enough down the drug discovery pipeline. Because of this, there are often not preapproved drug or treatment clinical trial protocols in place, ready to be implemented.

Innovations in Trial Design

In bioemergencies, the standard approach to generating evidence for informing medical practice may not be appropriate or feasible. There is growing interest in developing adaptive protocols that allow for flexibility and adaptability in study design through the use of ongoing data analysis and modeling to inform design structure. This approach has a twofold benefit of increasing the likelihood of obtaining usable, high-quality data from a variable and fast-paced study environment and reducing the cost-prohibitive price tag of traditional clinical trials.

In addition, trial networks that form around specific clinical areas of interest and capitalize on each other's existing research infrastructure are becoming increasingly common. They develop to share the burden of research infrastructure needs across multiple sites. Often, this is accomplished with common master or model protocols, central IRBs, central biorepositories, and innovative approaches to sharing resources [15].

Specimen Collection for Research Purposes

When conducting clinical research, it may be necessary to collect biospecimens from human subjects. Specimens may be collected for clinical purposes and used to inform a research study or may be collected specifically for research purposes. The Common Rule governs the collection of biological specimens from any living subject; in addition specific states and organizations may have their own rules regarding human samples. Specimen collection, retrieval, and practices will vary depending on type of research activity, nature of the specimen, and particular infectious disease of the patient. For example, a serum sample of a highly viremic Ebola virus disease patient will be addressed and handled differently than the nasal swab of a patient with an unidentified influenza-like illness. There are several best practice guidance documents regarding the handling of research specimens. For more information, see the laboratory chapter of this text (Chap. 6).

Storage and Future Use of Specimens and Data

Once collected, there is an option to store and maintain biological specimens and associated data for unspecified future use in a biorepository. A biorepository is a collection of any human biological materials and/or data that is intended to be used for research purposes, even if the purposes are not yet known. The data and specimens may be identifiable or de-identified (either coded or anonymous). This process is especially useful in a bioemergency as patients able to be enrolled in research studies may be sporadic or small in numbers. The OHRP provides specific guidance on the use of identifiable existing specimens and data in their guidance on Coded Private Information or Specimens Use in Research [2, 16–18].

Repository activities involve three components: the collection, storage, and distribution of materials and/or data. Specific IRB approval and continuing oversight are required for banking of specimens. The decision to store specimens and data for future use should be approved in advance of their collection. Federal regulation requires separate consent for the storage of biological materials. Subsequent research use of identifiable materials may require additional informed consent from subjects. Alternately, the consent provided at the time of banking of the information or specimens may have been sufficiently descriptive of what the stored specimen would be used for (i.e., consent to use may have already been obtained) that no additional permission would be required. Finally, separate consent for use of the specimens could be waived if the research is minimal risk, will not affect the rights and welfare of the subjects, and the research not be practicably carried out if additional consent were required (under HHS regulations) 45 CFR 46.116(d).

It is the responsibility of the investigator to maintain and protect human subjects records and specimens, and the resulting data, until they are properly destroyed. Federal regulations require research data to be retained for at least 3 years after the completion of the research [3]; however, many institutions have minimum amounts of time for keeping data upon completion of the research, so it is important to be aware of local requirements for both storage and (if necessary) appropriate destruction of data (and specimens.) As long as the researcher can guarantee that research data are secure, they can be kept indefinitely.

Participant Privacy

As noted above, collaboration is necessary for effective research in many bioemergencies as often times the disease may be rare and cases may be sporadic, particularly early in the emergency. This creates unique challenges around protecting the privacy of human subjects, particularly given the high level of media attention surrounding these events. For example, during the 2014–2016 Ebola virus disease outbreak, there was public awareness of the names of the few individuals treated in the USA. While formal measures for protecting and maintaining patient privacy should always be followed, they may not be sufficient in this context, and awareness of this is critical to reducing the risk of inadvertent participant identification [18–20].

Dissemination of Research Findings

While the goal of research is to inform generalizable knowledge, research data may be critical to response in the context of an unfolding public health emergency. Although publishing data is vital to the research process, it may delay dissemination of findings and potential beneficial changes in clinical practice or public health actions. In the wake of the Ebola outbreak of 2014–2016, the World Health Organization issued a consensus statement noting the need for more efficient and effective sharing of data and results in public health emergencies. Following this, several journals made sweeping changes to improve researchers' ability to share data, without negatively impacting their ability to publish resulting manuscripts [21, 22].

When conducting research in bioemergencies, investigators should be cognizant of the need for both timely information sharing and publication of formal results. Conflict can arise among study team members regarding priority and approach to both of these areas, and discussion of a dissemination plan should occur early in the development of a research study whenever possible.

Conclusion

Researchers are responsible for maintaining the public's confidence and upholding this trust through appropriate conduct of research, and this is especially important in the role of clinician scientist. The stakes are particularly high in the context of a bioemergency, a setting with opportunities for conducting clinically novel and critical research but also considerable challenges. Affected populations are inherently vulnerable, and all aspects of conducting research in this emergency environment are challenging. Careful adherence to the high standards set for human subjects research helps to ensure that the rights and welfare of individuals are protected in bioemergencies and that all persons maintain trust in the research relationship and process.

References

1. Otto JL, Holodniy M, DeFraites RF. Public health practice is not research. Am J Public Health. 2014;104(4):596–602.
2. Human Subject Regulations Decision Charts [Internet]. HHS.gov. 2017 [cited 29 October 2017]. Available from: https://www.hhs.gov/ohrp/regulations-and-policy/decision-charts/index.html. eCFR — Code of Federal Regulations [Internet]. Ecfr.gov. 2017 [cited 29 October 2017]. Available from: https://www.ecfr.gov/cgi-bin/ECFR?page=browse
3. Protection of Human Subjects, 45 C.F.R. §46 (2009). [regulation on the Internet]. [cited 29 October 2017]. Available from: https://www.ecfr.gov/cgi-bin/text-idx?tpl=/ecfrbrowse/Title45/45cfr46_main_02.tpl.
4. Mack A, Choffnes ER, Sparling PF, Hamburg MA, Lemon SM, editors. Ethical and legal considerations in mitigating pandemic disease: workshop summary. In: National Academies Press. Washington, DC; 2007.
5. Protection of Human Subjects, 21 C.F.R. §50.23 (2017). [regulation on the Internet]. [cited 29 October 2017]. Available from: https://www.accessdata.fda.gov/scripts/cdrh/cfdocs/cfcfr/CFRSearch.cfm?fr=50.23.
6. Protection of Human Subjects, 21 C.F.R. §50.24 (2017). [regulation on the Internet]. [cited 29 October 2017]. Available from: https://www.accessdata.fda.gov/scripts/cdrh/cfdocs/cfcfr/CFRSearch.cfm?fr=50.
7. Investigational New Drug (IND) Application [Internet]. Fda.gov. 2017 [cited 29 November 2017]. Available from: https://www.fda.gov/Drugs/DevelopmentApprovalProcess/HowDrugsareDevelopedandApproved/ApprovalApplications/InvestigationalNewDrugINDApplication/default.htm.

8. Protection of Human Subjects, 21 C.F.R. §56.104c (2017). [regulation on the Internet]. [cited 29 October 2017]. Available from: https://www.accessdata.fda.gov/scripts/cdrh/cfdocs/cfcfr/CFRSearch.cfm?fr=56.104.
9. Emergency Use Authorization of Medical Products and Related Authorities Guidance for Industry and Other Stakeholders [Internet]. Fda.gov. 2017 [cited 29 November 2017]. Available from: https://www.fda.gov/downloads/EmergencyPreparedness/Counterterrorism/MedicalCountermeasures/MCMLegalRegulatoryandPolicyFramework/UCM493627.pdf.
10. Schopper D, Dawson A, Upshur R, Ahmad A, Jesani A, Ravinetto R, Segelid MJ, Sheel S, Singh J. Innovations in research ethics governance in humanitarian settings. BMC Med Ethics 2015;16(1):10.
11. Altevogt B, Wizemann T, Reeve M, editors. Enabling Rapid and Sustainable Public Health Research During Disasters: Summary of a Joint Workshop by the Institute of Medicine and the US Department of Health and Human Services. Chapter 4: Addressing Institutional Review Board Barriers to Health Research Implementation.Washington, DC: National Academies Press; 2015.
12. National Ebola Training and Education Center [Internet]. NETEC. 2017 [cited 29 October 2017]. Available from: https://netec.org
13. NCATS Streamlined, Multisite, Accelerated Resources for Trials (SMART) IRB Reliance Platform. National Center for Advancing Translational Sciences (NCATS). October 14, 2016. (Retrieved from: https://ncats.nih.gov/expertise/clinical/smartirb).
14. Lane HC, Marston HD, Fauci AS. Conducting clinical trials in outbreak settings: points to consider. Clin Trials. 2016;13(1):92–5.
15. Woodcock J, LaVange LM. Master protocols to study multiple therapies, multiple diseases, or both. N Engl J Med. 2017;377(1):62–70.
16. Coded Private Information or Specimens Use in Research, Guidance (2008) [Internet]. HHS.gov. 2008 [cited 29 October 2017]. Available from: https://www.hhs.gov/ohrp/regulations-and-policy/guidance/research-involving-coded-private-information/index.html.
17. Allen MJ, Powers ML, Gronowski KS, Gronowski AM. Human tissue ownership and use in research: what laboratorians and researchers should know. Clin Chem. 2010;56(11):1675–82.
18. Guidelines and Policies for the Conduct of Research in the Intramural Research Programs at the NIH [Internet]. oir.nih.gov. 2015 [cited 29 October 2017]. Available from: https://oir.nih.gov/sites/default/files/uploads/sourcebook/documents/ethical_conduct/guidelines-conduct_research.pdf.
19. Horn EJ, Moore HM. Overcoming challenges in the acquisition of biospecimens for rare diseases. Expert Opin Orphan Drugs. 2013;2(1):1–4.
20. Schopper D, Ravinetto R, Schwartz L, Kamaara E, Sheel S, Segelid MJ, Ahmad A, Dawson A, Singh J, Jesani A, Upshur R. Research ethics governance in times of Ebola. Public Health Ethics. 2017;10(1):49–61.
21. Dye C, Bartolomeos K, Moorthy V, Kieny MP. Data sharing in public health emergencies: a call to researchers. Bull World Health Organ. 2016;94(3):158.
22. Developing global norms for sharing data and results during public health emergencies [Internet]. World Health Organization. 2015 [cited 29 October 2017]. Available from: http://www.who.int/medicines/ebola-treatment/blueprint_phe_data-share-results/en/.

Behavioral Health Support for Patients, Families, and Healthcare Workers

16

David S. Cates, Paula G. Gomes, and Arthur M. Krasilovsky

Introduction

During the 2014–2016 Ebola outbreak in West Africa, over 850 healthcare workers contracted Ebola, and over 500 died [1]. These tragic numbers underscore the need for strict adherence to infection control precautions when caring for patients with Ebola and other diseases that are both highly infectious and potentially fatal. In addition to the use of personal protection equipment (PPE), such measures include source isolation of infected patients. In the process of confining infectious pathogens, however, it is essential that health systems do not overlook the psychological needs of patients nor that of the medical staff who care for them. This chapter is divided into two sections. The first explores the experiences of patients cared for in source isolation, highlighting the possible iatrogenic psychological consequences of treatment on a biocontainment unit. Strategies for mitigating the potentially harmful psychological effects of isolation are reviewed, including considerations for children. The second section considers the experiences of healthcare workers. The discussion outlines the psychological impact of treating infectious diseases, risk factors for emotional distress, and strategies to promote psychological well-being and resilience.

D. S. Cates (✉)
Behavioral Health, Nebraska Medicine/University of Nebraska Medical Center, Omaha, NE, USA
e-mail: DCates@nebraskamed.com

P. G. Gomes · A. M. Krasilovsky
Faculty Staff Assistance Program, Emory University, Atlanta, GA, USA

A. Hewlett, A. R. K. Murthy (eds.), *Bioemergency Planning*,
https://doi.org/10.1007/978-3-319-77032-1_16

Source Isolation of Patients

Psychological Consequences

Patients treated in specialized hospital infection control units are subject to the full range of stressors attendant to hospitalization on any medical-surgical floor, such as incomplete understanding of the illness and treatment, anxiety about the outcome, painful conditions or procedures, and being away from home [2]. Beyond these sources of stress, however, patients treated in dedicated isolation rooms face a variety of unique challenges, including confinement in a small space, reduced opportunities for interaction with others, and potential stigmatization. Indeed, while source isolation is an essential strategy for minimizing risk to healthcare workers as well as the broader community, research conducted over the past two decades suggests that infection control precautions involving isolation may have negative psychological consequences for patients. Compared to hospitalized patients who are not isolated, for example, patients treated in isolation for multidrug-resistant organisms (MDROs) and *Clostridium difficile* are at increased risk for symptoms of depression and anxiety [3–7]. The data suggest that symptoms are likely to emerge after 2–3 days of isolation and may intensify with increased length of treatment [3, 4, 6–10]. Of course, beyond the effects of isolation, patients with life-threatening infectious diseases such as Ebola are at risk for significant emotional distress due to the traumatic nature of the symptoms themselves, the prospect of dying, and having witnessed or cared for others who died from the disease [11].

The literature on the psychological effects of isolation includes numerous qualitative-phenomenological studies, typically using semi-structured interviews to elicit patients' perceptions and recommendations. In addition to studying patients in source isolation for MDROs and *C. difficile*, this body of work includes patients in protective isolation for immunocompromised states, such as bone marrow transplant recipients. Despite differences in the circumstances associated with source and protective isolation, the evidence points to similarities in patients' reactions, including reports of loneliness [12–16], boredom [13, 16, 17], and fear [12, 18, 19].

Patients in isolation have also described feeling neglected and abandoned [13, 15, 17, 18, 20], with some characterizing the experience as prisonlike [12, 14, 16, 17, 20–22]. In a study of 24 US and French *C. difficile* patients interviewed within 14 months of hospitalization, several described feeling like outcasts and prisoners, with one patient comparing the experience to a horror film in which a victim is kept in a pit [12]. In addition, patients in isolation may regress to lower levels of functioning [23], such as requesting help with tasks they can perform themselves, seeking attention [13], or behaving in an abusive manner toward staff [20].

Beyond the loneliness, boredom, fear, abandonment, and regression described by patients in both source and protective isolation, those isolated for infectious conditions have described feelings of stigmatization [13, 17, 18, 21, 24]. Such patients have also reported fear and guilt regarding the prospect of spreading the infection to others [21].

Despite these reports, not all patients react negatively to isolation [25, 26]. In fact, some patients report liking the privacy and quiet [12, 13, 15, 17]. It should also be recognized that treatment in an isolation unit for a highly infectious condition is an unusual experience that generally occurs with little time for preparation. Consequently, an increase in anxiety or depression does not necessarily indicate preadmission or post-discharge psychiatric illness.

Possible Causes of Negative Psychological Effects

One factor that may contribute to the negative psychological impact of isolation is the loss of control associated with confinement in a small space for an indeterminate length of time [4, 13, 19, 23, 27, 28]. Beyond restriction to their rooms, patients in isolation typically have little say regarding who enters the room, when they can be alone, what food is available, and which clothes they can wear. In addition, curtailment in meaningful activities, including opportunities for socialization with friends, family, and other patients, may play a role in the harmful psychological consequences of isolation [13, 16–18, 22]. More generally, diminished sensory stimuli, including a limited view of the rest of the hospital unit [29, 30] and reduced visual contact with others [13], might also contribute to the adverse effects of treatment in an isolation room. Furthermore, when infection control precautions include masks, even face-to-face interactions with staff provide less sensory input [17]. Indeed, Ebola patients at both Nebraska Medicine and Emory University described frustration with the lack of full face-to-face visual contact as well as minimal tactile connection with others. Patients in source isolation for infections have also reported that isolation hampered their recovery and physical rehabilitation [17, 21, 29]. Finally, for patients isolated due to infectious diseases, the rapid implementation of infection control precautions, often with inadequate explanation [25], may be an additional source of psychological distress [13, 24].

Mitigating the Potentially Harmful Effects of Isolation

Investigators have recommended a variety of strategies to reduce the potentially harmful effects of isolation [31]. However, there appear to be no controlled studies examining whether such interventions are effective. With this caveat in mind, the following sections present considerations for hospitals to reduce the risk of negative psychological consequences associated with isolation (Table 16.1). While some suggestions apply to virtually all biocontainment units, others depend on the physical structure of the unit as well as on hospital and unit policies and procedures. The recommendations are based on the available literature, in connection with the clinical experience of the Nebraska Medicine and Emory University infection control teams.

Table 16.1 Summary of strategies to reduce the adverse psychological effects of isolation

	Communication	Control	Physical environment	Staff-patient interaction
Considerations for all patients	Make empathic statement when first meeting patient	Encourage patient to plan daily routines	Clock and calendar	Encourage patient to express concerns
	Explain infection control precautions and rationale	Schedule times without interruption	Window to outdoors	Listen actively
	Provide opportunities for patient to ask questions	Identify and honor preferences regarding visitors	Window looking onto unit, with convex mirror for wider view	Ask clarifying questions
	Repeat information	Inform patients about activities and supplies	Calming pictures on wall	Share something about life outside of hospital
	Use verbal, written, and video-based formats	Problem solve around desired activities not readily available	Shelving for personal belongings	Write staff names on gowns
	Employ professional interpreters	Provide opportunities to practice religion	Pictures from home	Provide photographs and brief bios of caregivers
		Allow ordinary clothes	Telephone, television, and computer	Train staff on adverse effects of isolation and strategies to minimize them
		Permit visitors and staff to bring in home-cooked or restaurant food	Games and snacks readily available in room	Facilitate contact with family and friends
			Exercise equipment	

(continued)

Table 16.1 (continued)

	Communication	Control	Physical environment	Staff-patient interaction
Additional considerations for children	Adapt information to child's maturity level	Provide initial orientation to unit	Age-appropriate toys and crafts	Hands-on activities for expression of feelings
	Ask what child "knows" about the hospitalization	Maximize family contact; should be predictable	Child friendly decor	Time for play
	Limit and discuss media exposure	Communicate changes to visit schedule in advance	Family pictures	Opportunities for decision-making and participation in care
	Clarify misconceptions	Consider time for schoolwork in daily routine	Comfort toys from home	
	Coach parents to model confidence in care team and outcome	Ensure consistency and honesty regarding discharge date		

Consistent, Clear Communication

Numerous authors have highlighted the role of communication in the isolation experience, either inadequate communication leading to increased distress or thorough communication making the experience more bearable [24, 30, 32–35]. At the same time, a number of studies suggest that many patients hospitalized with contact precautions do not understand the reasons for the infection control measures [15, 21, 24, 25, 32], even when provided with verbal and/or written information [15, 21]. Thus, a foundational strategy for reducing the potentially harmful psychological effects of isolation is ensuring that patients understand what precautions will be followed and the reasons for their implementation [6, 7, 30, 32, 34, 35]. One obstacle to achieving this objective is the difficulty patients may have processing information when under emotional and physical stress [15].

To reduce the impact of stress on comprehension, B. Reynolds of the Centers for Disease Control and Prevention recommended making an empathic statement within 30 s of meeting the patient in order to calm strong emotions [36]. A lower level of emotional arousal, in turn, can help the patient process the rest of the interaction. Providers should also give patients opportunities to ask questions and should be prepared to repeat information, perhaps multiple times. Along with providing information on infection control practices in both verbal and written forms [30, 32], hospitals can use video and internet-based formats, which some patients prefer [37]. Verbal, written, or video-based material can also include content on normal reactions to isolation and basic coping skills. Finally, if care team members do not speak the patient's primary language, a professional interpreter is necessary and may require telephone or video conferencing to reduce the risk of exposure.

Giving Patients Control

As mentioned above, the loss of control experienced by patients in isolation is one likely reason for the negative psychological effects [4, 28]. Consequently, giving patients as much control as possible over the daily routine, visitors, physical layout of the room, available activities, and, when feasible, the treatment itself may help improve psychological well-being [13, 19, 28, 34]. The long stretches of downtime during hospitalization, for example, provide an opportunity for patients to take some control over the schedule. Toward that end, staff can encourage patients to plan daily routines, including times for reading, eating, bathing, watching television, exercising, making phone calls, and engaging in any hobbies that may be accessible during hospitalization [20, 38, 39]. When possible, such plans should include specific times without interruption [28], which can be empowering for patients who otherwise have little control over healthcare workers' entering and exiting the room. In a similar vein, identifying and honoring patient preferences regarding visitation from family and friends (in person or via audiovisual media) can also promote patient autonomy [30].

In addition, care team members should discuss with patients available activities and supplies [6, 14, 30, 32, 35] such as books, newspapers, and crafts and problem solve around activities of interest that are not available. For example, staff in the Nebraska Medicine Biocontainment Unit (NBU) arranged for one patient to have access to drawing supplies, a variety of books, and a harmonica with instructions for beginners, based on the patient's stated interests. A small budget to make such activities accessible can go a long way toward ameliorating the potential boredom, loneliness, loss of control, and regression experienced by many patients in isolation. It is also important to inquire about religious preferences and to provide opportunities for patients to practice their religions [28], which may include video or telephone contact with hospital chaplains or community clergy.

Other ways to increase patients' sense of control as well as normalcy include allowing them to wear ordinary clothes (e.g., sweatpants) rather than hospital gowns [35] and permitting friends and family to bring in food, which can also strengthen patients' connections to life outside of the hospital [36]. At both Emory and Nebraska Medicine, for example, patients appreciated staff members' efforts to deliver favorite foods from local restaurants. Finally, empowering patients to make even trivial decisions, such as where to place the tray table or whether to keep the lights on or off, can make a difference in their sense of control over an otherwise highly restrictive situation [39].

The Physical Environment

Characteristics of the physical environment may also play a role in patients' well-being during isolation. Ensuring that rooms have a clock and a calendar can help patients stay oriented to the time and the day. A window to the outdoors may also help orient patients to time and lessen the sense of claustrophobia [13, 18, 28, 30,

35, 39]. Furthermore, a window looking onto the unit can provide additional sensory input and decrease feelings of isolation [13, 17, 29–31, 39]. In this regard, hospitals might consider installing convex mirrors outside of isolation room windows in order to provide a more complete view of the unit.

Although hospital rooms are often small and crowded with equipment, finding a portion of the wall for a poster, such as a nature scene, can help make a sterile environment more visually interesting [28, 31]. Furthermore, adequate shelving to allow patients to store some of their belongings can help patients to personalize their surroundings [20, 35]. Such shelving might also be used to display pictures from home, which can reinforce in patients a sense of connection to their lives outside of the hospital [16, 39].

Also essential in keeping patients connected to the outside world are a telephone, television, tablet, and computer [18, 32, 33], which have the additional benefit of helping patients stay busy [35]. In addition, having games available can serve as a source of both distraction and socialization [16]. Moreover, keeping snacks in patient rooms, rather than requiring patients to depend on unit staff to deliver food, can increase patients' feelings of control and independence [20].

Another consideration is providing exercise equipment for patients in isolation. Nebraska Medicine's NBU, for example, has a compact exercise bicycle that can be stationed in patient rooms. In addition, patients at both Emory and Nebraska Medicine enjoyed using a foam ball and basketball net. The opportunity to exercise can encourage patients to structure their days and can facilitate physical rehabilitation and overall well-being.

Staff Interaction with Patients

For many patients, the physical isolation associated with contact precautions leads to social isolation at a time when increased social support proves particularly critical [14, 18, 22]. Hospital staff can play a role not only in facilitating contact with friends and family (see below) but also in establishing a supportive and validating interpersonal connection [6, 14, 28, 30]. Cohen et al. [16] refer to this latter responsibility as "physical caregiving with a positive presence." Key elements of such compassionate staff-patient interaction include encouraging patients to express their concerns, using active listening skills, asking clarifying questions, and conveying understanding. In addition, patients often appreciate hearing some details about staff members' lives outside of the hospital [28].

Because staff ID badges are not worn or covered by gowns pursuant to infection control procedures, biocontainment unit teams should consider alternative means by which patients can identify caregivers. At both Nebraska Medicine and Emory, for example, staff members write their names across their gowns. Chronicling his experience in isolation for multidrug-resistant tuberculosis, Mayho [20] suggests that patients receive photographs of team members since caregiver faces are obscured by masks. Including a brief biographical sketch along with staff pictures might increase patients' level of comfort with their healthcare providers. For some members of the team, such information may be available via the hospital's web-based provider profiles. Patients in the NBU expressed appreciation and a sense of relief on seeing provider faces unobstructed by PPE when directed to online profiles.

More generally, unit administrators should ensure that all staff members receive education on the potentially harmful psychological effects of isolation and ways to minimize them [7, 24, 31]. Such in-service training should include discussion of possible regressive and disruptive patient conduct in order to inoculate team members against the natural tendency to take such behavior personally and help them develop constructive responses.

Family Contact

Contact with family members is for many isolated patients a crucial source of social and emotional support, as well as an invaluable connection to the outside world [14, 28]. Family contact may also play an important role in alleviating the feelings of boredom, loneliness, and neglect often described by patients in isolation [18, 30, 31, 35]. Such contact may be arranged through a secure audiovisual connection. At both Nebraska Medicine and Emory University, a separate room for family members provides a private and comfortable space for family to gather and to communicate via video with their loved one.

Children in Isolation

Psychological Consequences for Children

Although a detailed discussion of the psychological impact of isolation precautions on children is beyond the scope of this chapter, it should be noted that the potentially harmful effects on adults described above may also apply to children. In their qualitative study of children hospitalized with suspected or probable severe acute respiratory syndrome (SARS), Koller et al. [40] found that isolation precautions significantly disrupted family-centered care, leading to distress among children, their parents, and the healthcare workers who attended to them. The young patients in this sample experienced sadness, loneliness, and worry. More generally, hospitalized children may show anxiety, depression, homesickness, fear, withdrawal, and sleep disruption [41–44], depending in part on their age and personality characteristics. Hospitalized children have also been reported to display regression, anger, aggression, and demanding behavior [41, 43].

Interventions for Children

The strategies described above for mitigating the potentially harmful effects on adults also apply to children, though they must be tailored to the child's development level (see Table 16.1). For example, while frequent information sharing by the care team is important for pediatric patients [40–43], healthcare workers and parents should present information at a level consistent with the patient's intellect and maturity so as not to overwhelm the child [41]. In this regard, asking children what they "know" about their hospitalization and isolation is an effective strategy to uncover misapprehensions, such as a belief that they did something wrong or that they are being punished. Likewise, children's exposure to media coverage of the infection should be limited and discussed to process what the child heard and to clarify misconceptions [40]. Finally, coaching parents to model confidence in the care team and optimism about the outcome of treatment is particularly important for children, who may look to their parents for cues regarding the competence of their providers and the seriousness of their conditions [42].

As with adults, active listening to encourage expression of feelings is essential. However, some children may be more apt to express themselves through writing, playing, or drawing. For such children, hands-on activities, such as making a book about their experiences, might prove helpful. More generally, hospitalized children need opportunities to play, whether formal sessions with designated "child life" staff, informal play with care providers or family members, or by themselves. Beyond providing a distraction, play can help children communicate, process, and master distressing emotions and experiences related to their isolation [41]. Thus, access to a range of age-appropriate toys and crafts, along with television, video, and other media, is essential. Similarly, room décor should be child-oriented [41].

As discussed with regard to adults, establishing structured routines, including time for schoolwork if the child is healthy enough [45], may be especially important for children's emotional well-being. When feasible, an initial orientation to the unit, including an introduction to daily routines along with viewing staff photographs, can increase children's sense of predictability and control. Furthermore, consistency and honesty regarding possible discharge dates are important in order to maintain trust [42]. In addition, pediatric patients' participation in their own care and decision-making, even concerning seemingly trivial matters, can help with adjustment to hospitalization [43].

Maximizing contact with family members is perhaps the most critical factor in reducing the potentially harmful effects of isolation on pediatric patients, particularly younger children [40–43]. Contact with family members should be predictable and any changes to the visit schedule communicated in advance [42]. The decision whether or not to allow parents at the bedside must be made on a case-by-case basis with careful consideration of the risks and benefits [46]. When parents cannot physically be in the room, regular and predictable contact using technology, such as a cell phone or web-based media, is essential [40, 42, 47, 48]. In addition, pictures of family, comfort toys from home, and activities that foster connection with family, such as writing letters, can help [42, 43]. Healthcare workers may also become temporary "substitute family" for children in isolation [40, p. 55].

Family Members

Family members of critically ill patients may experience a range of stressors related to uncertainty about the outcome of the illness, economic hardship, and role disruption (e.g., as a parent, employee, or spouse) [47, 49]. Also common are feelings of helplessness, loneliness, anxiety, and sadness, as well as anger at or resentment toward the care team or even the patient [40, 48]. Furthermore, family members might experience guilt about feeling angry. They may also feel guilty about their inability to help and being healthy while their loved one is ill [48]. Family members of patients with infectious diseases may face additional hardships, including worry about other relatives' contracting the virus, feeling deprived of contact with their loved ones due to the isolation precautions, and stigma and social isolation within their communities [40, 47, 50]. Additionally, when a child is the patient, parents may experience "overwhelming fear" regarding their child's isolation and separation [47, p. 402].

The family's ability to cope with the above stressors can impact the patient's well-being and recovery. Consequently, hospitals should consider strategies to minimize the stress experienced by family members and to maintain their emotional, physical, and spiritual health. Bulling et al. [36] cogently summarize approaches that care teams can adopt to support families of patients in isolation. Perhaps the most important is regularly providing information, including specifics regarding the patient's condition, the treatment, and any risks to the family [18, 36, 40, 48–51]. Furthermore, making arrangements to keep family members informed when they are away from the hospital can help reduce anxiety and encourage needed breaks [36, 40, 47]. Additionally, providing information about normal family reactions, including fear of contracting the illness themselves, might help allay concerns among loved ones that their feelings are abnormal and can assuage any guilt about such reactions. When concerned family members include young children, suggesting concrete activities that promote children's connections to their loved ones in isolation can help. For example, children can draw pictures to decorate the hospital room or help prepare care packages.

Care team members can also encourage families to use existing support networks. At the same time, staff can empower family members to limit interaction with others when necessary, including turning off cell phones and disconnecting from social media, particularly in cases garnering media attention [36, 49]. In this regard, hospital staff can encourage family members to remain vigilant regarding how they share information within their support network, as personal social media posts can quickly become news when unit activations are covered by the press.

When treating patients with Ebola, Nebraska Medicine's NBU provided families with a concierge nurse who arranged for transportation, lodging, meals, regular meetings with the medical team, and video conferencing with patients. This proved to be an essential resource for decreasing the stress experienced by family members, all of whom were from out of town. Along with their physical and psychological needs, evaluating families' religious and spiritual needs, and facilitating access to clergy or hospital chaplains when indicated, may be critical for some families [36, 49]. Finally, when family members display significant emotional distress or difficulty coping that interferes with their ability to care for themselves or their loved ones, referral to a behavioral health provider should be considered [36].

Role of the Behavioral Health Specialist

In her review of strategies for minimizing the negative effects of isolation on patients with MRSA, Jones [31] recommended psychological screening of all patients. This approach may prove useful for biocontainment units as well. Behavioral health providers can introduce themselves as members of the biocontainment unit team, assess for mental health problems, and offer information on common psychological reactions. Additionally, behavioral health specialists can use psychological first aid principles and techniques to help patients connect with social supports, reinforce use of existing coping resources, and assist with problem-solving [52]. If necessary, behavioral health providers can suggest ways for patients to structure their time as well as teach specific coping skills, such as deep breathing, progressive muscle relaxation, mindfulness, and healthy thinking.

For some patients, ongoing supportive therapy may be indicated. Behavioral health providers should also be prepared to treat patients with adjustment disorders or acute stress disorder, particularly those with potentially fatal infections such as Ebola. Such patients may be severely stressed or traumatized by the symptoms of the illness itself as well as having witnessed or cared for others who were critically ill and who may have died [11, 53]. Providers can also make referrals for psychopharmacological intervention when necessary. In addition, some hospital facilities may consider the use of a palliative care team to address behavioral health concerns depending, in part, on the patient's health status.

Behavioral health providers may meet with patients via an audiovisual connection to minimize the risk of exposure to infectious diseases. Video consultation has the additional benefit of allowing patients to see the provider's face, which would otherwise be obscured by PPE. Another important role for the behavioral health specialist is providing support to the biocontainment unit team, which is the focus of the following section.

Behavioral Health Considerations for Healthcare Workers

In recent years, global and local health systems mobilized to develop comprehensive response protocols for patients with emerging infectious diseases, including severe acute respiratory syndrome (SARS), Middle East respiratory syndrome coronavirus (MERS-CoV), Ebola virus, and Lassa fever. To meet the growing demand for skilled healthcare workers required by these outbreaks, healthcare systems developed multifaceted responses including specialized assignments within hospitals, military and humanitarian deployments, and volunteer efforts (locally and globally). In response, healthcare workers (HCWs) answered the call to service.

Many studies have examined the effects of responding to these infectious disease crises on HCWs assigned to specialized hospital units or deployed internationally. In this regard, investigators have stressed the importance of active planning to promote and support the well-being of HCWs as systems prepare organizationally to manage and contain emerging infectious diseases. This section outlines the

Table 16.2 Challenges faced by HCWs in biocontainment units [55–58]

Personal challenges	Work-related challenges
Fear of contracting illness	Difficulties with proper use of personal protective equipment (PPE) and infection control protocols
Concerns for safety of family and friends	Lack of organization and role clarity
Isolation from family	Lack of resources
Communication and pressure from family members, lack of support	Altered standards of care and ethical conflicts
Continued pressure to justify work commitment	Safety and security
Sense of loss of control	Community response
Stigmatization, lack of appreciation	Isolation from regular unit colleagues
Directed negative community response toward individual and family members	Sense of being underappreciated
Fatigue and limited rest time	Team pressure to save patients
Feeling misunderstood	Witnessing the death of patients
Personal pressure to succeed in care of patients	Challenging team dynamics; managing stress and emotions effectively
Self-doubt, PTSS	Lack of sustained organizational support
Reentry stress at home	Loss of executive sponsorship
	Stress with reentry to regular unit
	Team engagement from frontline to ancillary staff

[a]At the Emory SCDU and Nebraska Medicine NBU, HCWs experienced some of these challenges while caring for Ebola and Lassa fever patients

psychological impact of treating infectious diseases on HCWs, risk factors for emotional distress, and organizational strategies to promote psychological well-being and resilience.

Challenges and Psychological Consequences for HCWs

There is notable consistency in the literature on the challenges faced by HCWs in voluntary, assigned, and deployed positions on biocontainment units [54–56]. Table 16.2 presents the most frequent personal (self, family, community) and work-related (job tasks, team, work location) challenges reported by HCWs treating a mixture of infectious diseases [55–57]. For some HCWs in hospital settings facing the epidemics of SARS and MERS-CoV, there were additional challenges due to caring for colleagues as patients within their facilities and being forcibly quarantined when workers developed symptoms [57, 59, 60].

Healthcare workers practicing in highly stressful, life-threatening environments are likely to experience psychological distress and are at risk of developing post-traumatic stress symptomatology (PTSS) and a variety of psychiatric morbidities [54, 55, 57, 61–66]. These outcomes, along with staff absenteeism while working in such settings [64, 66, 67], are more likely to occur in connection with the challenges outlined in Table 16.2 [54–56, 64, 65]. Symptoms may appear shortly after the outbreak is under control rather than during its height [54]. Emotional distress and psychiatric morbidity generally decrease over time, though relapse may occur, especially for those with preexisting mental health conditions and re-exposure to additional infectious disease outbreaks. For some HCWs, chronic posttraumatic stress disorder, depression, and anxiety were clinically diagnosed 2 years after exposure [54].

Risk Factors for Psychological Distress

As indicated above, it is evident that HCWs experience some level of emotional distress, ranging from moderate levels of worry [67] to posttraumatic stress symptoms and mental illness [54, 60, 65, 67–69]. A recent comprehensive review and meta-analysis of peer-reviewed articles published between January 2000 and December 2014 reveals that HCWs who are deployed and/or perceive themselves at a heightened risk of infection are more likely to experience psychological distress, insomnia, alcohol/drug misuse, PTSS, depression, and anxiety [54]. Additional risk factors for psychological distress and mental illness include longer duration of high-risk exposure, younger age, being single, not living with family, fewer years of work experience, lower education, and lower household income [54]. Other important factors to consider are previous history of psychiatric illness, availability of emotional support, and employer-sponsored resilience training [68, 70–73]. These findings underscore the importance of prevention and intervention strategies to promote self and team care among HCWs.

Strategies for Individual and Family Resilience

Given the significant psychological risks of biocontainment work environments, it is imperative that healthcare systems integrate behavioral health support, resilience training, and continuing education into the development plan for biocontainment teams. Engaging in comprehensive preparedness that addresses psychosocial challenges, as well as technical biocontainment training, can increase the skills and confidence of HCWs, reduce the negative psychological impact, enhance communication and collaboration, and reinforce the organization's commitment to supporting staff [54, 63, 66]. In particular, the evidence supports the design of an intervention model that targets individual and family resilience, in addition to organizational leadership, to reduce the risk of psychological distress for HCWs caring for patients with infectious diseases [54, 57, 59, 63, 70, 74, 75].

Individual Resilience

Individual resilience is the ability to reduce the effect of a stressful life event, cope with adversity, or bounce back [74]. Below are strategies that care teams can adopt to promote resilience in HCWs who volunteer or are assigned to work on biocontainment unit teams:

- Schedule individual information sessions with prospective staff members to review the roles, expectations, responsibilities, challenges, and rewards prior to the formal interview process. In addition to providing an opportunity to address any required occupational health clearance considerations, the session should prompt individuals to think about past experiences working in challenging roles as well as any history of PTSS or PTSD [66].
- Discuss with prospective staff members the motivating factors that contribute to their pursuit of these high-risk assignments. Frequently cited motivations include the uniqueness of the opportunity, professional interest, excitement about contributing to the field, desire to do something different, recognition, enhancing the reputation of the facility, improving one's CV, and helping others [55, 56]. HCWs from Emory University and Nebraska Medicine shared similar motivations for work with their biocontainment units.
- During the initial exploration phase of working in a high-risk environment, discuss with HCWs their suitability and preparation for the work. Verify that staff members have a full understanding of what will be involved from clinical, technical, psychosocial, and community perspectives.
- Recruit a behavioral health consultant to assist unit leadership in addressing concerns and questions that may emerge during recruitment of prospective staff.
- Include a resilience measure in preassignment health assessments to identify those at risk for developing a mental health disorder during or after the assignment [54].
- During the initial orientation and training, incorporate a module on behavioral health considerations, including strategies for strengthening resilience. This is currently part of the training sponsored by the National Ebola Training and Education Center (NETEC). Educating teams about behavioral health risks related to working in biocontainment units reinforces the importance of self and team care while reducing the stigma associated with psychological distress.
- Consider peer support training, which is a frequently cited approach to enable active monitoring for PTSS [66]. The trauma risk management (TRiM) program, for example, is used by military forces, media companies, and diplomatic organizations. Another model is psychological first aid, which can be implemented to support staff with early signs of distress [66, 74].
- Provide ongoing education sessions related to symptom recognition, effective coping strategies, and stigma reduction.
- Integrate a behavioral health specialist (BHS) into the biocontainment team. The BHS can provide on-site support (individual and group) utilizing a psychological first aid approach. This strategy serves as a bridge for HCWs to access a mental health clinician, who can connect staff to other providers as needed. Both the Emory Special Communicable Diseases Unit (SCDU) and Nebraska Medicine NBU have incorporated psychological support services through the Faculty Staff Assistance Program (FSAP) and the Behavioral Health division, respectively. Ideally, the BHS should attend regular team training sessions so that staff is familiar and comfortable with the provider. When the unit is activated, the BHS should spend time in the staff break room to maintain visibility and access.

- Establish a mentorship or "buddy" system that pairs new staff with more experienced colleagues [59].
- Provide access to individual counseling and support groups to manage psychological distress, including secondary traumatization [58, 62, 69]. These services can be provided by internal resources such as occupational health, employee assistance programs (EAP), or hospital behavioral health departments.
- Arrange debriefing sessions when critical incidents occur. These services can be offered by the BHS or spiritual health providers to support HCWs with processing complex feelings about the biocontainment work, especially once patients are discharged or pass away.

Family Resilience

Family resilience involves the potential for recovery, repair, and growth in families facing serious life challenges [76]. For HCWs treating infectious diseases, family resilience is essential, as family members are often affected by the work choices and experiences of their loved ones. Moreover, HCWs need to feel confident that their families are coping effectively while they are engaged in special assignments. Accordingly, health systems should develop strategies to foster resilience in family members before, during, and after special assignments [57, 76]. A variety of approaches are summarized below.

- Schedule a pre-deployment general information session about unit activation procedures, staff member roles, equipment, responsibilities, and stressors. Address fears, risks, and coping strategies as part of the session [55, 64]. One study found that this approach assisted HCWs with the transition back to their usual jobs after completion of their assignments [70].
- Encourage families to develop a "family plan" to address how roles and responsibilities, such as carpooling, grocery shopping, and meal preparation, might be altered should the HCW face quarantine or increased work hours.
- Provide additional sessions to update families on the unique aspects of particular unit activations. This may be offered online, in person, or via conference call.
- Arrange periodic group support sessions for HCWs' families. In addition, an annual family outing or picnic provides family members an opportunity to develop relationships that can reduce the isolation they may feel during an activation.
- Alert family members to the possibility of media interest in unit activations, and discuss potential consequences of sharing information with friends, employers, colleagues, and community contacts.
- Upon unit deactivation, schedule family debriefing sessions to enhance knowledge, respond to inquiries, and promote family resilience.

Organizational Leadership

Organizational leaders have a significant impact on the psychological well-being of HCWs navigating high-risk, trauma-exposed work environments. In particular, leaders who provide supportive engagement, a clear vision, and feedback and recognition to HCWs increase the probability of a successful biocontainment unit activation [70]. Lack of leadership support and effective communication, on the other hand, can leave workers feeling unappreciated, isolated, and devalued [70].

- Develop a strategy team including representatives from key functional areas to oversee resilience and well-being initiatives for staff working with emerging infectious diseases [63].
- Recruit senior leaders to meet with HCWs to communicate the organizational commitment to the biocontainment unit team. These sessions can reinforce to staff that hospital leaders appreciate and value the specialized work in which they are engaged.
- Offer leadership training to supervisors to ensure that they have the skills needed to build and maintain a healthy work culture. Key topics include effective communication, conflict management, team building, and stress management.

Future Directions

Research Needs

Although dozens of investigators have studied the psychological effects of source isolation as a component of contact precautions for infectious diseases, significant gaps in our understanding remain. Future research should examine the individual, family, illness, treatment, and environmental factors that predict who will be most impacted by source isolation. In addition, prospective research with baseline and multiple follow-up periods could help clarify the relationship between duration of isolation and patient distress. Such research should also evaluate patients after discharge to explore possible long-term psychological sequelae of various infectious diseases and their treatment. Preliminary evidence shows that, for example, 4–7 months after discharge, patients treated for Ebola continue to have psychological or cognitive symptoms, including sleep disturbance, short-term memory loss, and depression or anxiety [54]. Furthermore, randomized trials of interventions proposed to mitigate the impact of isolation are necessary, along with efforts to determine which interventions are best suited for which patients. Moreover, as most of the studies on source isolation involve patients with MDROs, more work is needed to examine the psychological impact of isolation in the context of treatment for potentially deadly infections, such as Ebola.

Research aimed at identifying the individual characteristics and skills that predict effective stress management and resilience during and after deployment is needed to help institutions identify and recruit prospective staff members for specialized infection control assignments. Furthermore, additional research on interventions designed to promote resilience before, during, and after deployment is necessary. Such studies can guide healthcare systems in providing the most effective support possible to protect the workforce from psychological distress and mental illness. While there is a tendency for investigators to focus primarily on nurses and physicians because of their frontline patient care responsibilities, ancillary team members are also vulnerable to the psychological distress inherent in the work with emerging infectious diseases. These positions may include patient transport staff, lab workers, pharmacists, facility management professionals (especially those handling biohazardous waste), and administrative assistants. From recruitment and training to activation and debriefing, it is essential to provide our workforce evidence-based, comprehensive behavioral health services to prevent, treat, and manage the negative psychological effects of high-stress and high-risk biocontainment unit activations.

References

1. World Health Organization. WHO Ebola situation report. 6 May 2015.
2. Kotrotsiou E, Theodosopoulou H, Papathanasiou I, Dafogianni C, Raftopoulos V, Evagelos K. How do patients experience stress caused by hospitalization and how do nurses perceive this stress experienced by patients? A comparative study. ICU Nurs Web J. 2001;7:1–17.
3. Catalano G, Houston S, Catalano M, Butera A, Jennings S, Hakala S, et al. Anxiety and depression in hospitalized patients in resistant organism isolation. South Med J. 2003;96(2):141–5.
4. Gammon J. Analysis of the stressful effects of hospitalisation and source isolation on coping and psychological constructs. Int J Nurs Pract. 1998;4:84–96.
5. Davies H, Rees J. Psychological effects of isolation nursing (1): mood disturbance. Nurs Stand. 2000 Mar 29;14(28):35–8.
6. Soon M, Madigan E, Jones K, Salata R. An exploration of the psychologic impact of contact isolation on patients in Singapore. Am J Infect Control. 2013;41:e111–3.
7. Tarzi S, Kennedy P, Stone S, Evans M. Methicillin-resistant Staphylococcus aureus: psychological impact of hospitalization and isolation in an older adult population. J Hosp Infect. 2001;49(4):250.
8. Day H, Morgan D, Himelhoch S, Young A, Perencevich E. Association between depression and contact precautions in veterans at hospital admission. Am J Infect Control. 2011;39:163–5.
9. Wassenberg M, Severs D, Bonten M. Psychological impact of short-term isolation measures in hospitalised patients. J Hosp Infect. 2010;75:124–7.
10. Day H, Perencevich E, Harris A, Gruber-Baldini A, Himelhoch S, Brown C, et al. Depression, anxiety, and moods of hospitalized patients under contact precautions. Infect Control Hosp Epidemiol. 2013;34(3):251–8.
11. Van Bortel T, Basnayake A, Wurie F, Jambai M, Koroma A, Muana A, et al. Psychosocial effects of an Ebola outbreak at individual, community and international levels. Bull World Health Organization. 2016;94(3):210–4.
12. Guillemin I, Marrel A, Lambert J, Beriot-Mathiot A, Doucet C, Kazoglou O, et al. Patients' experience and perception of hospital-treated Clostridium difficile infections: a qualitative study. Patient. 2014;7:97–105.
13. Oldman T. Isolated cases. Nurs Times. 1998;94(11):67–70.
14. Biagioli V, Piredda M, Alvaro R, De Marinis M. The experiences of protective isolation in patients undergoing bone marrow or haematopoietic stem cell transplantation: systematic review and metasynthesis. Eur J Cancer Care. 2017;26(5):1–13.
15. Newton J, Constable D, Senior V. Patients' perceptions of methicillin-resistant Staphylococcus aureus and source isolation: a qualitative analysis of source-isolated patients. J Hosp Infect. 2001;48:275–80.
16. Cohen M, Ley C, Tarzian A. Isolation in blood and marrow transplantation. West J Nurs Res. 2001;23(6):592–609.
17. Knowles H. The experience of infectious patients in isolation. Nurs Times. 1993;89(30):53–6.

18. Barratt R, Shaban R, Moyle W. Behind barriers: patients' perceptions of source isolation for Methicillin-resistant Staphylococcus aureus (MRSA). Aust J Adv Nurs. 2011;28(2):53–9.
19. Gammon J. The psychological consequences of source isolation: a review of the literature. J Clin Nurs. 1999;8:13–21.
20. Mayho P. Barrier grief. Nurs Times. 1999;95(31):24–5.
21. Skyman E, Sjostrom H, Hellstrom L. Patients' experiences of being infected with MRSA at a hospital and subsequently source isolated. Scand J Caring Sci. 2010;24:101–7.
22. Farsi Z, Nayeri N, Negarandeh R. The coping process in adults with acute leukemia undergoing hematopoietic stem cell transplantation. J Nurs Res. 2012;20(2):99–108.
23. Denton P. Psychological and physiological effects of isolation. Nursing. 1986;3(3):88–91.
24. Madeo M. Understanding the MRSA experience. Nurs Times. 2001;97(30):36–7.
25. Gasink L, Singer K, Fishman N, Holmes W, Weiner M, Bilker W, et al. Contact isolation for infection control in hospitalized patients: is patient satisfaction affected? Infect Control Hosp Epidemiol. 2008;29(3):275–8.
26. Livorsi D, Kundu M, Batteiger B, Kressel A. Effect of contact precautions for MRSA on patient satisfaction scores. J Hosp Infect. 2015;90:263–6.
27. Abad C, Fearday A, Safdar N. Adverse effects of isolation in hospitalised patients: a systematic review. J Hosp Infect. 2010;76:97–102.
28. Gaskill D, Henderson A, Fraser M. Exploring the everyday world of the patient in isolation. Oncol Nurs Forum. 1997;24(4):695–700.
29. Kennedy P, Hamilton L. Psychological impact of the management of methicillin-resistant staphylococcus aureus (MRSA) in patients with spinal cord injury. Spinal Cord. 1997;35(9):617.
30. Ward D. Infection control: reducing the psychological effects of isolation. Br J Nurs. 2000;9(3):162–70.
31. Jones D. How to reduce the negative psychological impact of MRSA isolation on patients. Nurs Times. 2010;106(36):14–6.
32. Rees J, Davies H, Birchall C, Price J. Psychological effects of source isolation nursing (2): patient satisfaction. Nurs Stand. 2000;14(29):32–6.
33. Cheng H, Qin L, Tee H. An exploratory study on the isolation experience of patients with haematological disorders. Singapore Nurs J. 2008;35(1):15–23.
34. Barratt R, Shaban R, Moyle W. Patient experience of source isolation: lessons for clinical practice. Contemp Nurse. 2011;39(2):180–93.
35. Madeo M. The psychological impact of isolation. Nurs Times. 2003;99(7):54–5.
36. Bulling D, Zagurski R, Hoffman S. Behavioral health guidelines for medical isolation. Lincoln, NE: University of Nebraska–Lincoln, Public Policy Center; 2007.
37. Gudnadottir U, Fritz J, Zerbel S, Bernardo A, Sethi A, Safdar N. Reducing health care-associated infections: patients want to be engaged and learn about infection prevention. Am J Infect Control. 2013;41:955–8.
38. Coenson C, Dimsdale J. Psychiatric liaison on a bone marrow transplantation unit. Gen Hosp Psychiatry. 1994;16:131–4.
39. Collins C, Upright C, Aleksich J. Reverse isolation: what patients perceive. Oncol Nurs Forum. 1989;16(5):675–9.
40. Koller D, Nicholas D, Goldie R, Gearing R, Selkirk E. When family-centered care is challenged by infectious disease: pediatric health care delivery during the SARS outbreaks. Qual Health Res. 2006;16(1):47–60.
41. Shields L. The psychosocial care of children in the perioperative area. In: Shields L, editor. Perioperative care of the child: a nursing manual. Chichester, UK: Wiley-Blackwell; 2010. p. 13–22.
42. Thurber C, Walton E, Council on School Health. Preventing and treating homesickness. Pediatrics. 2007;119(1):192–201.
43. Salmela M, Salantera S, Aronen E. Coping with hospital-related fears: experiences of preschool-aged children. J Adv Nurs. 2010;66(6):1222–31.
44. Meltzer L, Mindell J. Pediatric sleep. In: Roberts M, Steele R, editors. Handbook of pediatric psychology. 4th ed. New York: Guilford; 2009. p. 491–507.

45. Hostert P, Motta A, Enumo S. Coping with hospitalization in children with cancer: the importance of the hospital school. Estud Psicol. 2015;32(4):627–39.
46. Davies H, Byington C, Committee on Infectious Diseases. Parental presence during treatment of Ebola or other highly consequential infection. Pediatrics. 2016;138(3):e1–6.
47. Chan S, Leung D, Chui H, Tiwari A, Wong E, Wong D, et al. Parental response to child's isolation during the SARS outbreak. Ambul Pediatr. 2007;7(5):401–4.
48. Wochna V. Anxiety, needs, and coping in family members of the bone marrow transplant patient. Cancer Nurs. 1997;20(4):244–50.
49. Wu J, Mu P, Tsay S, Chiou T. Parental experience of family stress during hematopoietic stem cell transplantation of pediatric patients in germ-free isolation in Taiwan. Cancer Nurs. 2005;28(5):363–71.
50. Sengupta A, Rand C, Perl T, Milstone A. Knowledge, awareness, and attitudes regarding methicillin-resistant Staphylococcus aureus among caregivers of hospitalized children. J Pediatr. 2011;158(3):416–21.
51. Briggs J, Milstone A. Changes over time in caregivers' knowledge, attitudes, and behaviors regarding methicillin-resistant Staphylococcus aureus. J Pediatr. 2011;158(6):1039.
52. Brymer M, Jacobs A, Layne C, Pynoos R, Ruzek J, Steinberg A, et al. Psychological first aid: field operations guide. 2nd ed. Washington, DC: National Child Traumatic Stress Network and National Center for PTSD; 2006.
53. Mohammed A, Sheikh T, Gidado S, Abdus-salam I, Adeyemi J, Olayinka A, et al. Psychiatric treatment of a health care worker after infection with Ebola virus in Lagos, Nigeria. Am J Psychiatry. 2015;172(3):222–4.
54. Vyas K, Delaney E, Webb-Murphy J, Johnston CS. Psychological impact of deploying in support of the U.S. response to Ebola: a systematic review and meta-analysis of past outbreaks. Mil Med. 2016;181(11/12):e1515–31.
55. Gideon J, Harper S, Williams P, Ostrom S, Bredbere S, Amlôt R, et al. How to support staff deploying on overseas humanitarian work: a qualitative analysis of responder views about the 2014/15 West African Ebola outbreak. Eur J Psychotraumatol. 2016;7:30933.
56. Gershon R, Dernehl L, Nwankwo E, Zhi Q, Qureshi K. Experiences and psychosocial impact of West Africa Ebola deployment on US health care volunteers. PLoS Curr. 2016 Sept 21;8:1–24.
57. Hall R, Hall R, Chapman M. The 1995 Kikwit Ebola outbreak: lessons hospitals and physicians can apply to future viral epidemics. Gen Hosp Psychiatry. 2008;30(5):446–52.
58. Lee S, Juang Y, Su Y, Lee H, Lin Y, Chao C. Facing SARS: psychological impacts on SARS team nurses and psychiatric services in a Taiwan general hospital. Gen Hosp Psychiatry. 2005;27(5):352–8.
59. Maunder R, Lancee W, Balderson K, Bennett J, Borgundvaag B, Evans S, et al. Long-term psychological and occupational effects of providing hospital healthcare during SARS outbreak. Emerg Infect Dis. 2006;12(12):1924–32.
60. Khalid I, Khalid T, Qabajah M, Barnard A, Qushmaq I. Healthcare workers emotions, perceived stressors and coping strategies during a MERS-CoV outbreak. Clin Med Res. 2016;14(1):7–14.
61. Bitanihirwe B. Monitoring and managing mental health in the wake of Ebola. Ann Ist Super Sanita. 2016;52(3):320–2.
62. Styra R, Hawryluck L, Robinson S, Kasapinovic S, Fones C, Gold W. Impact on health care workers employed in high-risk areas during the Toronto SARS outbreak. J Psychosom Res. 2008;64(2):177–83.
63. Aiello A, Khayeri M, Raja S, Peladeau N, Romano D, Leszcz M, et al. Resilience training for hospital workers in anticipation of an influenza pandemic. J Contin Educ Health Prof. 2011;31(1):15–20.
64. Sim K, Chong P, Chan Y, Soon W. Severe acute respiratory syndrome-related psychiatric and posttraumatic morbidities and coping responses in medical staff within a primary health care setting in Singapore. J Clin Psychiatry. 2004;65(8):1120.

65. Wu P, Fang Y, Guan Z, Guan Z, Fan B. The psychological impact of the SARS epidemic on hospital employees in China: exposure, risk perception and altruistic acceptance of risk. Can J Psychiatry. 2009;54:302–11.
66. Greenberg N, Wessely S, Wykes T. Potential mental health consequences for workers in the Ebola regions of West Africa – a lesson for all challenging environments. J Ment Health. 2015;24(1):1–3.
67. Goulia P, Mantas C, Dimitroula D, Mantis D, Hyphantis T. General hospital staff worries, perceived sufficiency of information and associated psychological distress during the A/H1N1 influenza pandemic. BMC Infect Dis. 2010;10:322.
68. Lancee W, Maunder R, Goldbloom D. Prevalence of psychiatric disorders among Toronto hospital workers one to two years after the SARS outbreak. Psychiatr Serv. 2008;59(1):91–5.
69. Matsuishi K, Kawazo A, Imai H, Ito A, Mouri K, Kitamura N, et al. Psychological impact of the pandemic (H1N1) 2009 on general hospital workers in Kobe. Psychiatry Clin Neurosci. 2012;66(4):353–60.
70. Brooks S, Dunn R, Sage C, Amlot R, Greenberg N, Rubin G. Risk and resilience factors affecting the psychological wellbeing of individuals deployed in humanitarian relief roles after a disaster. J Ment Health. 2015;24(6):385–413.
71. McMahon S, Ho L, Brown H, Miller L, Ansumana R, Kennedy C. Healthcare providers on the frontlines: a qualitative investigation of the social and emotional impact of delivering health services during Sierra Leone's Ebola epidemic. Health Policy Plan. 2016;31(9):1232–9.
72. Greenberg N, Langston V, Iverson A, Wessely S. The acceptability of trauma risk management within the UK armed forces. Occup Med. 2011;61:184–9.
73. Greenberg L, Langston V, Everitt B, Iverson A, Fear N, Jones N, et al. A cluster randomized controlled trial to determine the efficacy of Trauma Risk Management (TriM) in a military population. J Trauma Stress. 2010;23(4):430–6.
74. Maunder R, Leszcz M, Savage D, Adam M, Peladeau N, Romano D, et al. Applying the lessons of SARS to pandemic influenza: an evidence-based approach to mitigating the stress experienced by healthcare workers. Can J Public Health. 2008;99(6):486–8.
75. Folkman S, Greer S. Promoting psychological well-being in the face of serious illness: when theory, research and practice inform each other. Psychooncology. 2009;9:11–9.
76. Walsh F. Family resilience: strengths forged through adversity. In: Walsh F, editor. Normal family processes: growing diversity and complexity. 4th ed. New York: Guilford; 2012. p. 399–427.

Index

A. Hewlett, A. R. K. Murthy (eds.), *Bioemergency Planning*,
https://doi.org/10.1007/978-3-319-77032-1

Printed and bound by PG in the USA